Current Practices in Ophthalmology

Series Editor
Parul Ichhpujani, Department of Ophthalmology
Government Medical College and Hospital
Chandigarh, India

This series of highly organized and uniform handbooks aims to cover the latest clinically relevant developments in ophthalmology. In the wake of rapidly evolving innovations in the field of basic research, pharmacology, surgical techniques and imaging devices for the management of ophthalmic disorders, it is extremely important to invest in books that help you stay updated. These handbooks are designed to bridge the gap between journals and standard texts providing reviews on advances that are now part of mainstream clinical practice. Meant for residents, fellows-in-training, generalist ophthalmologists and specialists alike, each volume under this series covers current perspectives on relevant topics and meets the CME requirements as a go-to reference guide. Supervised and reviewed by a subject expert, chapters in each volume provide leading-edge information most relevant and useful for clinical ophthalmologists. This series is also useful for residents and fellows training in various subspecialties of ophthalmology, who can read these books while at work or during emergency duties. Additionally, these handbooks can aid in preparing for clinical case discussions at various forums and examinations.

Daisy Shu • Rohan Bir Singh
Parul Ichhpujani
Editors

Current Advances in Optometry

Springer

Editors
Daisy Shu
School of Optometry and Vision Science,
Faculty of Medicine and Health
University of New South Wales (UNSW)
Sydney, NSW, Australia

Parul Ichhpujani
Department of Ophthalmology
Government Medical College and Hospital
Chandigarh, India

Rohan Bir Singh
Department of Ophthalmology, Harvard
Medical School
Schepens Eye Research Institute of Mass
Eye and Ear
Boston, MA, USA

ISSN 2523-3807 ISSN 2523-3815 (electronic)
Current Practices in Ophthalmology
ISBN 978-981-97-8139-3 ISBN 978-981-97-8140-9 (eBook)
https://doi.org/10.1007/978-981-97-8140-9

This Springer imprint is published by the registered company Springer Nature Singapore Pte Ltd.
The registered company address is: 152 Beach Road, #21-01/04 Gateway East, Singapore 189721, Singapore

Preface

We welcome our readers to the fascinating subject of optometry and its dynamic landscape, which will definitely shape the way you practice today as well as in the future. This book delves into the intricate science and artistry behind vision care, exploring the marvels of the intricate mechanisms that provide us sight. Whether you are an optometry graduate, a seasoned optometrist, or an ophthalmologist seeking to deepen your understanding, or simply an enthusiast curious about the novel wonders of visual assessment and rehabilitation, this book will illuminate and inspire you.

Optometry is a discipline at the intersection of ophthalmology, physics, and technology, continuously evolving with advancements in science and innovation. Optometry is more than just diagnosing and correcting refractive errors. It encompasses a holistic approach to eye health, encompassing preventative care, disease management, and rehabilitation. Throughout this book, we emphasize the importance of comprehensive eye examinations, early detection of eye conditions, and the role of optometrists as primary eye care providers.

Within these pages, we endeavour to capture not only the recent advances in the field of optometry but also the established fundamentals. Our exploration begins with the differences in global optometry practices, advances in the management of ocular surface disorders and cornea, as well as glaucoma. From there, we venture into the realms of diagnostics, examining the tools and techniques used to assess colour vision and tailoring precise prescriptions for contact lenses, vision therapy, and low vision aids. We also delve into the relevant clinical trials for optometrists, novel ocular drug delivery modalities, and the application of artificial intelligence in optometry.

As we journey through these pages, it is essential to remember that optometry is not merely a profession but a calling—a commitment to safeguarding one of our most precious senses, enriching lives, and empowering individuals to experience the world with clarity and confidence.

We extend our heartfelt gratitude to all the contributors, researchers, educators, and clinicians whose dedication and expertise have enriched the field of optometry and made this book possible. We earnestly hope that this book serves as a valuable resource, inspiring readers to explore, learn, and contribute to the remarkable field of optometry.

With curiosity as our compass and knowledge as our guide, let us embark on this illuminating journey into the world of optometric practices.

Chandigarh, India — Parul Ichhpujani
Boston, MA, USA — Rohan Bir Singh
Sydney, NSW, Australia — Daisy Shu

Acknowledgments

Alone we can do so little, together we can do so much.–Helen Keller

I would like to extend my deepest gratitude to all those who have contributed to the creation of this book, from the authors who shared their expertise to the editorial team who worked tirelessly to ensure its quality and accuracy. It is my sincere hope that this book will serve as a beacon of inspiration and a valuable resource for those seeking to explore the advances in the realm of optometry.

Parul Ichhpujani

Contents

Differences in Optometry Practices Across the Globe

Shivani Majithia and Sahil Thakur

Key Points

- The World Council of Optometry provides the four categories of scopes of optometry practices.
- These include the optical technology services (OT), visual function services (VF), ocular diagnostic services (ODx), and ocular therapeutic services (OTx).
- Level 4 services are predominantly concentrated in regions like the UK, USA, and Oceania, while the majority of global practices are Level 2 or Level 3.

1 Introduction

In the realm of eye care, two distinct yet interdependent professions, ophthalmology, and optometry, play pivotal roles in safeguarding and enhancing our most treasured sense: vision. Ophthalmology stands as the medical specialization tasked with the diagnosis and treatment of eye diseases, with a focus on surgical interventions. Optometry, on the other hand, focuses on the assessment and correction of refractive errors and the prescription of corrective lenses. The collaboration between these two professions is integral to providing comprehensive eye care, but their individual roles and practices vary considerably across the globe. Understanding these differences is crucial, as it not only sheds light on the evolution of healthcare practices but also illuminates the socio-cultural and economic factors shaping the delivery of eye care services.

S. Majithia
Education and Professional Services, Essilor Luxottica, Singapore
e-mail: shivani.majithia@essilor.com

S. Thakur (✉)
Singapore Eye Research Institute, Singapore, Singapore

Medical Affairs, Mediwhale, Seoul, South Korea

D. Shu et al. (eds.), *Current Advances in Optometry*, Current Practices in Ophthalmology, https://doi.org/10.1007/978-981-97-8140-9_1

This chapter embarks on journey through the diverse landscapes of optometry practices across different regions, aiming to uncover the nuances that shape the way we perceive and treat vision-related concerns. As we traverse the landscape of optometry practices, we will meticulously examine one country from each major global region to highlight the intricate tapestry of practices, regulations, and challenges that characterize the optometric field. By delving into these regional disparities, we aim to enrich the understanding of how cultural, societal, and economic contexts shape the provision of eye care services. From the educational paths leading to optometry licensure to the scope of services offered by optometrists, we will scrutinize the unique facets that define each country's optometry practices. Through this chapter, we hope to paint a comprehensive picture of the variations in optometry practices across the world. By doing so, we aspire to foster a deeper appreciation for the diverse ways in which societies address visual health and refractive needs, ultimately highlighting the need for global collaboration to ensure that the gift of sight is cherished and preserved universally.

The world is a tapestry of cultures, economies, and healthcare systems, each contributing to the diverse fabric of optometry practices. Optometry, as a profession dedicated to preserving and enhancing visual health, manifests in varied ways across different continents and regions. This section of this chapter thus embarks on a journey across the globe, exploring the distinct optometry practices that have evolved in response to unique societal, cultural, and economic contexts.

1.1 World Council of Optometry

The World Council of Optometry (WCO) defines the scope of optometry as, "a healthcare profession that is autonomous, educated, and regulated (licensed/registered), and optometrists are the primary healthcare practitioners of the eye and visual system who provide comprehensive eye and vision care, which includes refraction and dispensing, detection/diagnosis and management of disease in the eye, and the rehabilitation of conditions of the visual system [1]." This definition plays a pivotal role in delineating the parameters of optometry, characterizing it as an independent, knowledge-intensive healthcare discipline that operates within a regulated framework of licensure and registration. The WCO offers several guidelines, consensus documents and educational resources that can be used by stakeholders interested in the profession [2, 3]. The WCO has outlined its 2021–2024 strategic plan, "One Voice of Optometry" that has outlined four themes: inspiring optometric education; integrating optometry in broader health sector; membership support and growth; and future planning and collaborations with international bodies like WHO and IAPB [3]. In addition to these advocacy activities, the WCO also provides a competency based model of Scope of Practice in Optometry to assist states and countries around the world to reconcile the variations in the scope of optometric practice internationally. The competency model includes four categories of services that provide a vertical ladder for individuals seeking to expand their career. The WCO defines four categories of practice types [3]. They are outlined in Table 1.

Table 1 Four categories of scopes of practice by the world council of optometry

Level 1	Optical Technology Services (OT)	This includes management and dispensing of ophthalmic lenses, ophthalmic frames and other ophthalmic devices that correct defects of the visual system
Level 2	Visual Function Services (VF)	This includes investigation, examination, measurement, recognition, and correction/management of defects of the visual system. *The practitioners at Level 2 are considered to be optometrists*
Level 3	Ocular Diagnostic Services (ODx)	This includes investigation, examination and evaluation of the eye and adnexa, and associated systemic factors, to detect, diagnose, and manage disease
Level 4	Ocular Therapeutic Services (Otx)	This includes use of pharmaceutical agents and other procedures to manage ocular conditions/disease

The WCO currently has 36 country members and is the leading global body for advocacy, education, policy development and humanitarian outreach for optometrists [4]. For the subsequent chapter, we will use the four levels of practice to categorize the optometry services in different global regions.

2 Optometry Practices in Different Global Regions

2.1 North America: United States (Level 4)

United States (US), boasts of a well-established optometry practice deeply integrated into the healthcare systems. Optometrists are educated to diagnose and treat various eye conditions, prescribe corrective lenses, and provide pre- and post-operative care. The optometrists in US embark on a comprehensive educational journey, commencing with 4 years of undergraduate studies followed by 4 years in Optometry school to get Doctor of Optometry (OD) degree, with some pursuing an additional fifth year of specialized training. Recently some institutions also offer combined degrees with MPH, MBA, and PhD [5]. There are 24 schools and colleges of optometry under the Association of Schools and Colleges of Optometry (ASCO)—23 are in the continental US, and one is in Puerto Rico. The regulatory bodies and professional associations play pivotal roles in shaping education and licensure requirements [5, 6]. The regulations are however governed by state laws and are thus amenable to constant practice updates [6]. In certain states like Louisiana optometrists can perform several laser procedures, including YAG capsulotomy, peripheral iridotomy, and selective laser trabeculoplasty [7]. The readers are thus advised to look at online resources to review the clinical and therapeutic scope of optometrists in the US [8]. Currently optometrists in all states have oral medication authority and can treat glaucoma topically [8]. They can also remove ocular foreign bodies and order blood panels or imaging studies such as CT or MRI. In some states they can perform refractive procedures and minor lid surgery [8]. Optometrists in US are also required to obtain continuing education credit hours to maintain licensure. Organizations like the American Optometric Association

(AOA) provide regularly updated, high-quality, evidence-based clinical practice guidelines for common eye diseases [9, 10]. As per the Bureau of Labour Statistics employment estimates 40,640 optometrists in the US, earning a mean annual wage of $133,100, with most employed in optometry co-practices [11]. Therefore, in summary, the US boasts a well-established and highly specialized field of optometry, delivering top-tier diagnostic and treatment services for eye health.

2.2 Europe: Europe (Level 3) and United Kingdom (Level 4)

In Europe, optometry practices vary from country to country. The European Council of Optometry and Optics (ECOO) represents the interests of optometrists and opticians across Europe. The ECOO represent more than 150,000 opticians and optometrists from 22 European Union (EU) countries. The European Diploma accredited by the ECOO is set at the Bachelor level in European Higher Education and provides a qualification defined for optometric practice at WCO Category 3 [12]. The ECOO also provides online resources on education, advocacy and professional conduct for use for professionals [13]. The United Kingdom (UK), however, has a system where optometrists are trained to diagnose and treat a range of eye conditions, prescribe medications, and refer patients to ophthalmologists when necessary. They are regulated by the General Optical Council (GOC) through the Opticians Act 1989, and they are distinct from medical practitioners. Registration with the GOC is mandatory for practicing optometry in the UK [14]. The optometrists complete a 4-year undergraduate honors degree followed by a 1-year internship. Successful completion of assessments and supervised practice qualifies them to register with the GOC and potentially join the College of Optometrists. Members of the College of Optometrists can use the designation MCOptom. The College of Optometrists also provides clinical management guidelines [15] for 62 diseases and drug formulary [16] of 71 drugs that the optometrists can prescribe. To sum up, the United Kingdom also showcases a firmly established and extensively specialized domain of optometry, providing exceptional diagnostic and therapeutic solutions for maintaining ocular health. Table 2 presents the standards of practice recommended by different organizations, the GOC provides the most detailed 19 standards in that list [18].

2.3 Asia: India (Levels 2 and 3)

Asian countries like India reflect a diverse spectrum of optometry practices. In India, optometry has been rapidly evolving as a standalone profession with a growing emphasis on primary eye care and refractive correction. Optometrists in India are trained to diagnose and manage common eye conditions, often working in rural and urban settings. The Indian Optometry Federation described three types of optometry cadres: the trained ophthalmic assistants/technicians (2 year), the diploma trained optometrists (2 year) and the degree trained optometrists (4 year) [21]. The Ministry for Health and Family Welfare, Government of India has

Table 2 The standards of practice/code of conduct for optometrists

Organization	Country	Standards
World Council of Optometry [17]	Global	1. Keep your patients' eye, vision, and general health your first priority 2. Respect the rights and dignity of patients regarding their health care decisions 3. Advise your patients whenever consultation with, or referral to, another optometrist or other healthcare professional is appropriate 4. Ensure confidentiality and privacy of patients' health and other personal information 5. Strive to ensure that all people have access to eye and vision care 6. Advance your professional knowledge and skills 7. Maintain your practice in accordance with professional health care standards 8. Promote ethical and cordial relationships with all members of the health care community 9. Uphold the dignity, honor, and integrity of the optometric profession
General Optical Council [18]	United Kingdom	1. Listen to patients and ensure that they are at theheart of the decisions made about their care 2. Communicate effectively with your patients 3. Obtain valid consent 4. Show care and compassion for your patients 5. Keep your knowledge and skills up to date 6. Recognize, and work within, your limits of competence 7. Conduct appropriate assessments, examinations, treatments, and referrals 8. Maintain adequate patient records 9. Ensure that supervision is undertaken appropriately and complies with the law 10. Work collaboratively with colleagues in the interests of patients 11. Protect and safeguard patients, colleagues, and others from harm 12. Ensure a safe environment for your patients 13. Show respect and fairness to others and do not discriminate 14. Maintain confidentiality and respect your patients' privacy 15. Maintain appropriate boundaries with others 16. Be honest and trustworthy 17. Do not damage the reputation of your profession through your conduct 18. Respond to complaints effectively 19. Be candid when things have gone wrong
Optometry Council of India [19][a]	India	1. Respect your patient 2. Provide accessible and suitable setup 3. Maintain privacy and confidentiality 4. Provide relevant and evidence-based management 5. Provide appropriate referrals

(continued)

Table 2 (continued)

Organization	Country	Standards
Australian Health Practitioner Regulation Agency [20]	Australia	1. Put patients first—Safe, effective, and collaborative practice 2. Aboriginal and Torres Strait islander health and cultural safety 3. Respectful and culturally safe practice for all 4. Working with patients 5. Working with other practitioners 6. Working within the healthcare system 7. Minimizing risk to patients 8. Professional behavior 9. Maintaining practitioner health and wellbeing 10. Teaching, supervising, and assessing 11. Ethical research

The codes and standards are available on the official website of the concerned regulator and advisory bodies
[a]The general guideline from the Optometry Council of India have been adopted from the section A of the best practice in standards of Optometry handbook available at the official website [19]

provided the model curriculum for Bachelors (4 years) and Masters of Optometry (2 years) courses [22]. It also describes the job scope of optometrists in India. The scope fits into WCO Category 3 with additional provision to only use diagnostic medications, namely mydriatics and cycloplegics [22]. Recently, the National Commission for Allied & Healthcare Professionals Act, 2021 has been passed and optometry has been recognized as a profession in India [23]. The introduction of PhD programs in select institutions, such as the Elite School of Optometry in Chennai, has significantly broadened the prospects and horizons available to optometrists [24]. In summary, Indian optometry is thus poised to align with global counterparts in the collective pursuit of eliminating avoidable blindness and propelling advancements within various specialized realms of optometry. This transformation is underscored by recent legislative and regulatory reforms that have streamlined and fortified the profession's trajectory.

2.4 Africa: Botswana (Level 3)

The African continent presents a diverse range of healthcare challenges, influencing optometry practices. Progress is evident, especially with efforts toward a united African Union, yet significant health issues such as visual impairment and blindness often persist, due to refractive errors. Optometry thus emerges as a key solution to address vision impairment on the continent. There are about 17 institutions in 10 countries offering 14 fully accredited programs [25]. The programs include Diploma in Optometry, Bachelor of Optometry, and Doctor of Optometry degrees. However, meeting the demand for optometric professionals primarily requires establishing more institutions with uniform curriculum and standards. Significant challenges in staffing, infrastructure, and training resources also exist. One such example is Botswana, where the Botswana Optometrists Association (BOA) aims to act as the voice of optometrists [26]. Most optometrists are foreign trained and work in the private sector. The organization's main role is to advance optometry and eye healthcare through advocacy and support. It empowers optometrists in Botswana to excel in their profession, acting as their representative in engagements with government bodies, health councils, and relevant organizations [4]. By fostering professional growth and development, the organization also ensures high-quality care. It collaborates with the Botswana Health Professions Council for peer reviews and continuing education activity. Securing financial assistance and maintaining transparent communication with stakeholders, members, and the public are also integral functions. The organization also conducts regular eye camps, spectacle distribution and public education activities. Ultimately, the organization strives to enhance optometry in Botswana and undertakes all possible actions to achieve these goals [4, 26].

2.5 Oceania: Australia and New Zealand (Level 4)

In the Oceania region, Australia and New Zealand showcase comprehensive optometry practices. Optometrists in these countries are trained to diagnose, manage, and co-manage a variety of eye conditions. The Optometry Board of Australia is responsible for registering optometrists and students, establishing profession-related standards, managing complaints and investigations, evaluating overseas practitioners, and approving accreditation standards and courses [27]. The scope of optometry practice includes therapeutic prescribing, enabling optometrists to treat certain eye diseases. In the "Working Together for Better Eye Care" scope of optometry document, Optometry Australia recommends actions that can be implemented to better utilize the skills of optometrists to enhance patient access and increase the efficiency of Australia's eye health system [28]. Australia has a total of 6175 registered optometrists who are actively practicing. These professionals are spread across 1200 communities throughout the country. Their geographic distribution closely mirrors the overall population, although there are certain underserved areas in rural and remote regions. Among the optometrists, approximately 56% are women, and an estimated 72% fall under the age of 50, indicating a relatively youthful demographic profile [28, 29]. While optometrists in New Zealand are allowed to prescribe oral medications for eye conditions like infections, inflammation, and allergies, optometrists in Australia are limited to use of topical medications [28]. Advocacy groups are also campaigning for provision of intravitreal drug injection privileges along with greater role in national screening programs for chronic diseases like cataract, glaucoma, age related macular degeneration and diabetic retinopathy [28].

2.6 South America: Brazil and Colombia (Level 3)

Optometry practices in South America exhibit varying degrees of development [4]. In Brazil, optometrists have a prominent role in providing primary eye care and refractive correction, especially in underserved areas. Recently, optometry has been recognized in the Brazilian Supreme Court [30]. The Brazilian Council of Optics and Optometry (CBOO) is the main body for advocacy and formulating guidelines for optometrists. The goal of obtaining legal recognition is to reduce the societal impact due to diseases affecting the eye. This objective is pursued through a strategic approach that focuses on raising awareness and integrating optometrists into the public healthcare framework. Similarly in Colombia, the main advisory body is the Colombian Federation of Optometrists (FEDOPTO: En el Colegio Federación Colombiana de Optómetras) [31]. There are seven optometry schools in Colombia [32]. An intriguing report shed light on a significant disparity: although optometrists are legally permitted to conduct fundus and peripheral examinations with dilation, this practice remains infrequent and is predominantly carried out by ophthalmologists [33]. This underscores the urgency for advocacy and heightened awareness, aiming to harness the available workforce and mitigate the eyecare challenges faced in Latin America.

2.7 Middle East: Saudi Arabia and Dubai (Level 3)

The Middle East has a diverse range of optometry practices. In Saudi Arabia, the Saudi Society of Optometry (SSO) is the main advocacy organization [26]. The SSO plays a pivotal role in establishing a comprehensive scientific and educational platform that empowers optometrists to acquire knowledge and contribute effectively. It fosters health research in eye care, benefiting both the community and professionals in the field. The society also drives professional development, paving the way for a brighter future for the optometry profession in Saudi Arabia. By equipping optometrists with the skills to provide primary eye health care and combat blindness, the society significantly impacts public health. It leads efforts to enhance regulatory aspects within the optometry sector and establishes valuable collaborations with the private sector. Additionally, the society focuses on bolstering financial resources while upholding the best governance and institutional practices. Through its initiatives, the SSO promotes societal engagement, delivers health education, and ultimately elevates the public's perception of the optometry profession. As of 2021, there were a total of 1886 practicing optometrists in Saudi Arabia (64% male), with 45% practicing in Riyadh, according to the Saudi Commission for Health Specialties [34]. While in Dubai, an optometrist is defined as, 'a primary healthcare professional for the eye concerned especially with examining the eye for refractive error problems and prescribing spectacle lenses, contact lenses and low vision rehabilitation to correct these related problems' [35]. Thus, optometry services in Dubai mainly provide primary eye and vision care, eye examinations to detect vision problems and prescription of corrective lenses to correct those problems under Level 3 category of the WCO.

3 Summary

Currently, the majority of optometry practices worldwide fall within Level 2 or Level 3 categories as defined by the World Council of Optometry (WCO). Notably, Level 4 practices, which offer advanced ocular therapeutic services, are predominantly concentrated in regions like the UK, US, and Oceania. The future of optometry is anticipated to witness a growth in the number of optometrists providing ocular therapeutic services, spurred by promising outcomes from studies such as selective laser trabeculoplasty trials [36, 37]. However, this expansion requires the establishment of a standardized training scheme and robust governance measures to ensure the safe and effective delivery of these services across the profession.

References

1. Concept of Optometry: World Council of Optometry. 2020. https://worldcouncilofoptometry.info/concept-of-optometry. Accessed 27 Dec 2023.
2. Home: World Council of Optometry. 2023. https://worldcouncilofoptometry.info. Accessed 26 Dec 2023.
3. Resources: World Council of Optometry. 2022. https://worldcouncilofoptometry.info/resources. Accessed 27 Dec 2023.
4. Members: World Council of Optometry. 2023. https://worldcouncilofoptometry.info/our-members/#1597164269116-cdf0cb39-5831. Accessed 26 Dec 2023.
5. Association of Schools and Colleges of Optometry's (ASCO). Optometry programs admissions directory. Association of Schools and Colleges of Optometry, 2023. Accessed 27 Dec 2023.
6. American Optometric Association: Find Your State Board CE Requirements and Affiliate Contacts. 2023. https://www.aoa.org/member-center/doctors-of-optometry/find-your-state-board-or-affiliate-contact?sso=y. Accessed 27 Dec 2023.
7. Healio. Louisiana grants optometrists surgery privileges. 2014. https://www.healio.com/news/optometry/20140603/louisiana-grants-optometrists-surgery-privileges. Accessed on 27 Dec 2023.
8. Optometry scope of practice in the United States. Eyes On Eyecare 2022. https://eyesoneyecare.com/resources/optometry-scope-of-practice-united-states. Accessed 27 Dec 2023.
9. Clinical Practice Guidelines. American Optometric Association 2023. https://www.aoa.org/practice/clinical-guidelines/clinical-practice-guidelines?sso=y. Accessed 27 Dec 2023.
10. Gyawali R, Toomey M, Stapleton F, et al. Quality of 2019 American optometric association clinical practice guideline for diabetic eye care. Ophthalmic Physiol Opt. 2021;41(1):165–70.
11. Optometrists. US Bureau of Labour Statistics. 2023. https://www.bls.gov/oes/current/oes291041.htm. Accessed 25 Dec 2023.
12. European Diploma in Optometry | ECOO. 2023. https://ecoo.info/ecoo-accreditation-agency/european-diploma-in-optometry. Accessed 25 Dec 2023.
13. Resources | ECOO. European Council of Optometry and Optics, 2023.
14. Working in the United Kingdom | General Optical Council. General Optical Council, 2023.
15. Clinical management guidelines. The College of Optometrists. 2023. https://www.college-optometrists.org/clinical-guidance/clinical-management-guidelines.

16. Optometrists' formulary. The College of Optometrists 2023. https://www.college-optometrists.org/clinical-guidance/optometrists-formulary. Accessed 25 Dec 2023.
17. Optometrist code of conduct—World Council of Optometry. World Council of Optometry. 2020. https://worldcouncilofoptometry.info/optometrist-code-of-conduct. Accessed 25 Dec 2023.
18. Standards of practice for optometrists and dispensing opticians | General Optical Council. General Optical Council. 2023. https://optical.org/optomanddostandards.
19. Best practice standard: Optometry Council of India. Optometry Council of India. 2023. https://optometrycouncilofindia.org/best-practice-standard. Accessed 25 Dec 2023.
20. Shared code of conduct principles. Australian Health Practitioner Regulation Agency. 2023. https://www.ahpra.gov.au/Resources/Code-of-conduct/Resources-to-help-health-practitioners/Shared-Code-of-conduct-principles.aspx. Accessed 25 Dec 2023.
21. De Souza N, Cui Y, Looi S, et al. The role of optometrists in India: an integral part of an eye health team. Indian J Ophthalmol. 2012;60(5):401–5.
22. Optometry. Ministry of Health and Family Welfare. 2016. https://main.mohfw.gov.in/modelcurriculaforalliedandh/optometry.
23. The National Commission for Allied and Healthcare Professions Act, 2021. Ministry of Health and Family Welfare. 2021. https://main.mohfw.gov.in/newshighlights-46.
24. PhD Optometry. Elite School of Optometry: Shankar Nethralaya. 2023. https://www.eso.sankaranethralaya.org/ph-d-optometry.html.
25. Oduntan OA, Mashige KP, Kio FE, Boadi-Kusi SB. Optometric education in Africa: historical perspectives and challenges. Optom Vis Sci. 2014;91(3):359–65.
26. Website. Botswana Optometrists Association. 2023. https://boa.org.bw.
27. Statistics. Optometry Board of Australia. 2023. https://www.optometryboard.gov.au/about/statistics.aspx.
28. Scope of practice Optometry Australia. 2021. https://www.optometry.org.au/advocacy/issues-at-a-glance/optometric-scope-of-practice.
29. Our organisation Optometry Australia. 2022. https://www.optometry.org.au/about-us/our-organisation.
30. A new chapter in vision health in Brazil. The International Agency for the Prevention of Blindness. 2022. https://www.iapb.org/news/a-new-chapter-in-vision-health-in-brazil.
31. FEDOPTO—En el Colegio Federación Colombiana de Optómetras. 2023. https://fedopto.org.
32. List of Optometry schools—Colombia. 2023. https://www.liquisearch.com/list_of_optometry_schools/colombia.
33. Cevallos AA. Report on Colombia Optometry fellowship. 2022.
34. Alanazi MK, Almutleb ES, Badawood YS, et al. Perspectives and clinical practices of optometrists in Saudi Arabia concerning myopia in children. Int J Ophthalmol. 2023;16(2):267–73.
35. Regulation for optical center and optometry services. Dubai Health Authority. 2016. https://www.dha.gov.ae/uploads/112021/4c39c535-aeab-4315-a400-25129c734377.pdf.
36. Jones L, Konstantakopoulou E, Gazzard G. Selective laser trabeculoplasty (SLT) performed by optometrists for patients with glaucoma and ocular hypertension: a scoping review. BMJ Open Ophthalmol. 2021;6(1):e000611.
37. Konstantakopoulou E, Jones L, Nathwani N, Gazzard G. Selective laser trabeculoplasty (SLT) performed by optometrists-enablers and barriers to a shift in service delivery. Eye (Lond). 2022;36(10):2006–12.

Advances in Dry Eye Disease Diagnosis and Management

Rohan Bir Singh and Parul Ichhpujani

Dry eye disease (DED) is an inflammatory response of the eye caused by decreased production of tears, excessive evaporation of tears, or both [1]. It is a very common disorder in the USA and affects roughly 5% of adults nationally [1].

1 Epidemiology

DED is more common in people aged 50 and older and it is more common in women than in men [1]. Previous studies have found prevalence rates to vary from 5% to 34% worldwide [2]. The difference in prevalence between men and women is due to the effect of female hormones on the lacrimal and meibomian glands [3]. Other studies have estimated DED to affect 3.2 million women and 1.68 million men in the USA [4].

Global, population-based studies have found prevalence rates to vary from 5% to 50% around the world. This range is due to discrepancies in diagnostic criteria and what actually classifies as DED [3]. Additionally, for reasons that are unknown, prevalence is found to be higher in Asian populations as compared to White populations. Climate, geographic location, and environmental factors may explain these discrepancies [3]. DED prevalence also increases with age; as one gets older, tear production naturally decreases to an extent, and impaired tear production is the underlying issue behind DED [5].

R. B. Singh (✉)
Harvard Medical School, Boston, MA, USA
e-mail: rohan_singh@meei.harvard.edu

P. Ichhpujani
Department of Ophthalmology, Government Medical College and Hospital, Chandigarh, India

D. Shu et al. (eds.), *Current Advances in Optometry*, Current Practices in Ophthalmology, https://doi.org/10.1007/978-981-97-8140-9_2

The high prevalence of DED poses a great burden in terms of healthcare costs in the USA, especially as the population continues to age. The annual cost to the average patient with DED is estimated to be \$783 [2]. This equates to a \$384 million cost to the United States health care system every year [2]. Treatments for DED are continuing to evolve but as the population continues to age, prevalence levels will likely remain high nationwide.

2 Pathophysiology

DED is a caused by a variety of factors affecting the ocular surface and its tears. In a structurally functional eye, the ocular surface is kept lubricated by the lacrimal gland producing tears superiorly, and the meibomian sebaceous glands producing oils and lipids inferiorly [1]. Damage to any of these structures can precipitate the effects of DED. It is thought that external stressors on the ocular surface can trigger the body's natural immune response and thereby cause inflammation to these crucial structures of the eye [2]. These external stressors may be environmental, antigenic, infectious, or genetic. The inflammatory response of chemokines, cytokines, matrix metalloproteases, and the recruited T cells will then invade the ocular surface and its surrounding glands, rendering them nearly nonfunctional [2].

The normal tear film is composed of three main layers: the lipid layer, the aqueous layer, and the mucin layer [3]. The lipid layer is the most superficial layer and is made by the meibomian glands, which sit in the eyelid. The lipid component of the tear serves to decrease its evaporation, thereby, allowing for adequate lubrication [3]. Next, the job of the lacrimal gland, along with the accessory lacrimal glands, is to produce the middle, aqueous layer of the tear film. This layer is the thickest of the three layers and contributes to an overall film thickness of 2–5 μm [3]. Lastly, the base mucin layer is composed of glycoproteins, which are produced by goblet cells of the conjunctiva [3].

In DED, these structures, and therefore the integrity of the tears, are compromised. Inflammation of the lacrimal gland will lead to decreased production of the aqueous layer, resulting in a thinner tear film and a less hydrated eye [3]. If the meibomian glands are damaged due to inflammation, there will be no superficial lipid component of the tear film, making it vulnerable to increased evaporation [3]. These two mechanisms are the basis for the two subtypes of DED.

3 Subtypes

The two main subtypes of DED are defined as aqueous-deficient(ADED) or evaporative(EDED) [3]. Aqueous-deficient DED is due to reduced tear production, likely from an impaired lacrimal gland. Evaporative or hyperevaporative DED is due to impaired lipid production by the sebaceous meibomian glands, causing increased evaporation of the tear film. Of the patients with DED, about 10% have just the aqueous-deficient subtype. Most patients (over 80%) have either EDED or mixed ADED and EDED [2]. While the mechanism of the two subtypes differs, both mechanisms result in an impaired tear film, which leads to inadequate lubrication of the ocular surface. This decreased lubrication is the cause of the symptoms that patients with DED experience.

4 Symptoms

Many symptoms of DED can be vague and nonspecific; these include redness of the eye, burning or stinging, grittiness or the feeling of a foreign body in the eye, itchiness, and photophobia. These symptoms while nonspecific can greatly impair a patient's quality of life and their ability to carry out everyday activities comfortably; up to 60% of patients with DED report a reduced quality of life [2]. This can cause concurrent anxiety and/or depression for many patients. Prevalence of depression in patients with DED was roughly 5% higher when compared to the control group, one study found [2]. Additionally, DED can impair vision, affecting a patient's ability to drive or read, further impairing their quality of life and contributing to their depressive symptoms. Reduced reading speed and reduced driving reaction time, tested in a driving simulator, were both notable findings in patients with DED [2].

Additional findings in patients with DED include signs of impaired meibomian gland function, such as obstruction of the gland by a cloudy, granular excretion [2]. This must be removed by applying significant pressure on the lower eyelid where the gland is located. This impaired gland function may also result in blepharitis or meibomitis, or inflammation of the eyelid and the meibomian gland, respectively [2]. The inflammation of the ocular structures in DED may lead to damage of the ocular surface. This presents as small epithelial erosions on the ocular surface, also known as superficial punctate keratitis [2]. Often this is indicated by temporal conjunctival folds that are parallel to the lid margin.

5 Diagnosis and Treatment

DED can present similarly to allergies or certain infections, therefore, proper diagnosis is crucial to insure adequate treatment is provided. The first component of diagnosis is obtaining a detailed patient history about the symptoms, their severity, onset, and triggers as well as additional underlying health conditions and medications [2].

Next, examination of the eyelids can provide information about the condition and possible severity. Factors such as reduced blink rate (promoting tear evaporation), lid incongruity, and insufficient lid closure can also be seen. Examination of the lids themselves can provide insight into the functioning, or lack thereof, of the meibomian glands; a slit lamp can be used to visualize these in greater detail [2].

Another finding suggestive of DED is temporal lid-parallel conjunctival folds (LIPCOFs); this is a physical exam finding that is caused by increased friction between the eyelids and the surface of the conjunctiva [2]. This increased friction can be due to decreased lubrication from tears, therefore, indicating DED.

The slit lamp can also be used to visualize the ocular surface for signs of damage. One common dye, lissamine green, will stain damaged surface cells with a defective mucin layer, while fluorescein dye will highlight erosions in the conjunctiva and cornea [2]. Fluorescein will also stain tear film. In DED, significant staining in the region near the palpebral fissures will be seen [2].

Lastly, the tear film itself will be examined. The height of the tear film can be measured during a slit lamp examination and can be indicative of DED. The stability of the tear film is also measured via the tear film break-up time (TFBUT) [2]. A shorter TFBUT is often indicative of some underlying pathology [2]. Additional tests are present; however, they are subject to high variability and not often required to make the diagnosis [2].

Treatment for DED is primarily aimed at alleviating symptoms since it is a chronic disease. Patients should also be educated about their condition and certain aggravating factors such as dry air, smoke, or use of contact lenses [2]. Artificial tears are the main treatment for patients with DED; no studies have been done comparing different types of artificial tears, however. In general, it is known that artificial tears reduce ocular surface friction, improve tear film integrity, and increase patients' quality of life [2]. For patients with hyperevaporative DED, artificial tears containing a lipid component have been shown to improve tear film stability and meibomian gland function [2].

5.1 Tear Film Biomarkers

Tear-soluble factors such as cytokines and chemokines are the best surrogate markers of DED severity and can help in disease classification and treatment planning. Increased levels of cytokines, viz., interleukin-1β (IL-1β), IL-2, IL-4, IL-6, IL-9, IL-12, IL-17A, interferon-gamma (IFN-γ), tumor necrosis factor-alpha (TNF-α); chemokines (CCL2, CCL3, CCL4, C-X-C motif chemokine ligand 8; CXCL8); MMP-9, FGF, VEGF-A; soluble receptors (sICAM-1, sTNFR1), neurotrophic factors (NGF, substance P, serotonin) and IL1RA and reduced levels of IL-7, IL-17F, CXCL1, CXCL10, EGF, and lactoferrin have been found in DED [6].

Anti-inflammatory treatment is also recommended in patients with more severe forms of DED [2]. This is because the underlying mechanism of DED is thought to be an innate inflammatory response infiltrating the ocular surface structures. Chronic inflammatory insult to the ocular surface leads to the invasion of blood and lymphatic vessels into the cornea, which contributes to cellular trafficking [6]. During the inflammatory siege, granulocyte–macrophage–colony-stimulating factor (GM-CSF) secretion adds fuel to fire by the induction of monocytes/macrophages.

Corticosteroid eye drops are also available for patients with a more severe form of DED [2]. Again, this is likely due to reduced inflammation within the ocular surface structures that contribute to the DED symptoms. Lastly, certain immunomodulators and antimicrobial agents have shown some efficacy in reducing symptoms of DED due to their anti-inflammatory effects [2]. Further research is being done to understand the specific inflammatory pathways of DED, in hopes of developing more targeted treatment in the future [7].

6 Risk Factors

There are many potential risk factors for the development of DED, some more supported than others. Risk factors that are supported by a high level of evidence include age and female sex, as discussed before, post-menopausal hormone replacement therapy (HRT), and androgen insensitivity syndrome (AIS) [2]. Studies have shown that the meibomian gland dysfunction (MGD) occurs because of the hormones used in HRT and the lack of hormonal response in AIS [8, 9]. NOV03 (perfluorohexyloctane; under review with the US Food and Drug Administration [FDA]) is an emerging therapy for DED associated with MGD. This drug has shown significant improvements in both signs and symptoms [10].

Intense pulsed light (IPL) therapy, involving treatment over the eyelids, has emerged as a potential treatment for MGD by causing liquefaction of meibum, thrombosis of telangiectatic blood vessels in the eyelids, changes in meibomian gland architecture and photomodulation. A recent Cochrane review has shown that LipiFlow performs similarly to other commonly used DED treatment modalities as regards the DED signs and symptoms. A high level of bias was seen in the best available evidence, resulting in low certainty evidence [11]. In addition to the relatively high costs, IPL treatment may cause depigmentation or swelling of the periocular skin, eyelash loss or permanent iris transillumination defects.

Additional highly supported risk factors include anything that may affect the integrity of the ocular surface, such as collagen vascular disease, corneal refractive surgery, irradiation, vitamin A deficiency, and stem cell transplantation [2]. Patients using certain antihistamine drugs may also be at an increased risk of DED due to their mechanism of action, which decreases tear production as a side effect [12]. Lastly, for reasons that are unknown, patients with Hepatitis C are at a higher risk for developing DED [13].

Other possible risk factors for DED that are moderately supported by research include diabetes mellitus, isotretinoin, systemic chemotherapies, keratoplasty, sarcoidosis, HIV infection, and certain medications such as tricyclic antidepressants, selective serotonin reuptake inhibitors, and beta blockers [2]. Smoking, alcohol use, Botox injections, oral contraceptives, gout, and pregnancy are other possible risk factors for the development of DED, however, they are not well supported [2].

A point-of-care diagnostic kit, Bio-M Pathfinder (NovoMol-Dx, India, a customized version of the Ella™ Automated ELISA system, Bio-Techne®Corporation, Minnesota, USA) has been recently introduced in the Indian market for clinical use. This kit will help to identify the molecular status in patients with DED and additionally, help define the risk of development of DED in clinically healthy eyes planned for invasive procedures [6]. This will help in tailored management of these individuals ("personalized medicine").

7 Complications

Late stages of DED can progress to more severe symptoms, leading to ocular health complications. The consequences of the surface inflammation and the epithelial erosions can progress to conjunctival scarring, permanent epithelial defects, ulceration, or in very severe cases, corneal ulceration [2]. These complications may even lead to vision loss [3]. However, the severe complications listed above are very rare and often precipitated by underlying health issues and autoimmune syndromes. These include Stevens-Johnson Syndrome, Sjögren's Syndrome, xerophthalmia and vitamin A deficiency, and graft-versus-host disease [2].

8 Disease Progression and Future Direction

All in all, DED is a self-limited disease especially once symptoms are treated. Most patients see a reduction in symptoms as time progresses with the treatment, with no major progression of symptoms [4]. Some patients with a severe form of DED initially may report a worsening severity down the line, as well as patients with a lower level treatment course [4]. More research is needed to accurately track the progression of DED in patients with varying degrees of severity, along with the efficacy of different levels of treatment courses. Additionally, further research on the underlying inflammatory pathways triggered in DED must be conducted in order to develop more effective therapy for those with severe disease progression [6].

References

1. Walter K. What is dry eye disease? JAMA. 2022;328(1):84.
2. Messmer EM. The pathophysiology, diagnosis, and treatment of dry eye disease. Dtsch Arztebl Int. 2015;112(5):71.
3. Golden MI, Meyer JJ, Patel BC. Dry eye syndrome. St. Petersburg: StatPearls; 2023. Accessed 15 Dec 2023
4. Lienert JP, Tarko L, Uchino M, Christen WG, Schaumberg DA. Long-term natural history of dry eye disease from the patient's perspective. Ophthalmology. 2016;123(2):425.
5. Zhang X, Wang L, Zheng Y, Deng L, Huang X. Prevalence of dry eye disease in the elderly: a protocol of systematic review and meta-analysis. Medicine. 2020;99(37):E22234.
6. Kumar NR, Praveen M, Narasimhan R, Khamar P, D'Souza S, Sinha-Roy A, Sethu S, Shetty R, Ghosh A. Tear biomarkers in dry eye disease: progress in the last decade. Indian J Ophthalmol. 2023;71(4):1190–202.
7. Ling J, Chan BCL, Tsang MSM, et al. Current advances in mechanisms and treatment of dry eye disease: toward anti-inflammatory and immunomodulatory therapy and traditional Chinese medicine. Front Med (Lausanne). 2021;8:815075.
8. Cermak JM, Krenzer KL, Sullivan RM, Dana MR, Sullivan DA. Is complete androgen insensitivity syndrome associated with alterations in the meibomian gland and ocular surface? Cornea. 2003;22(6):516–21.
9. Schaumberg DA, Buring JE, Sullivan DA, Reza Dana MR. Hormone replacement therapy and dry eye syndrome. JAMA. 2001;286(17):2114–9.

10. Sheppard JD, Nichols KK. Dry eye disease associated with meibomian gland dysfunction: focus on tear film characteristics and the therapeutic landscape. Ophthalmol Ther. 2023;12(3):1397–418.
11. Pucker AD, Yim TW, Rueff E, Ngo W, Tichenor AA, Conto JE. LipiFlow for the treatment of dry eye disease. Cochrane Database Syst Rev. 2024;2(2):CD015448.
12. Katipoğlu Z, Abay RN. The relationship between dry eye disease and anticholinergic burden. Eye (Lond). 2023;37(14):2921–5.
13. Rajalakshmy AR, Malathi J, Madhavan HN, Bhaskar S, Iyer GK. Patients with dry eye without hepatitis C virus infection possess the viral RNA in their tears. Cornea. 2015;34(1):28–31.

Advances in Diagnosis and Management of Infectious Keratitis

Bharat Gurnani and Kirandeep Kaur

1 Introduction

Infectious keratitis (IK) is an acute or chronic infection of the cornea that poses a significant risk of visual impairment [1, 2]. It is a serious ocular condition that can result in corneal scarring, thinning, and perforation, potentially leading to blindness if not correctly managed. The etiology of IK is diverse, with bacterial, viral, fungal, and parasitic organisms all known to be causative agents [1]. The global burden of the disease is substantial, particularly in developing countries where access to health care is limited and risk factors, such as the use of traditional eye medications and poor hygiene practices, are prevalent [1, 3].

Current research on the occurrence of IK is limited, with most studies being over a decade old. The incidence rates of IK vary significantly based on geographic location and research methodology, ranging from 2.5 to 799 cases per 100,000 people annually [3–5]. This variation is particularly notable between high-income and low-income countries. For instance, past research indicated an incidence of 2.5–27.6 per 100,000 people per year in the USA and 2.6–40.3 per 100,000 people per year in the United Kingdom. Recent findings from a study in Nottingham, UK, align with these older studies, showing a steady incidence of 34.7 per 100,000 people per year from 2007 to 2019, suggesting a continuous presence of IK in developed countries [6].

Similarly, a study in Australia reported a lower incidence of 6.6 per 100,000 people per year between 2005 and 2015 [7]. However, these figures might be underestimates,

B. Gurnani (✉)
Cataract, Cornea, External Diseases, Trauma, Ocular Surface and Refractive Surgery, Gomabai Netralaya and Research Centre, Neemuch, India

K. Kaur
Cataract, Pediatric Ophthalmology, Strabismus and Neuro-Ophthalmology, Gomabai Netralaya and Research Centre, Neemuch, India

D. Shu et al. (eds.), *Current Advances in Optometry*, Current Practices in Ophthalmology, https://doi.org/10.1007/978-981-97-8140-9_3

as they were derived from cases requiring corneal scraping. Conversely, much higher rates of IK have been reported in less affluent countries. For example, South India recorded an incidence of 113 per 100,000 people per year, and Nepal reported a staggering 799 per 100,000 people per year [8]. The increased incidence in these areas can be attributed to factors like poor environmental and personal hygiene, lower educational levels, the prevalence of agricultural work, heightened risk of work-related corneal injuries, and limited access to sanitation and healthcare facilities [1].

The risk factors for infectious keratitis can be varied and are often associated with conditions that compromise the integrity or immune defense of the eye [9]. Some of the primary risk factors include contact lens use, ocular trauma, compromised immune function, exposure to contaminated water, poor eyelid hygiene, previous eye infections or surgeries, use of topical corticosteroids, dry eye syndrome, wearing decorative contact lenses, and environmental factors [10]. Addressing these risk factors through proper eye care, hygiene, and caution in potentially hazardous environments can significantly reduce the likelihood of developing infectious keratitis [2]. The diagnosis of infectious keratitis is primarily clinical but requires a high index of suspicion, especially in individuals presenting with risk factors such as contact lens use, recent ocular trauma, pre-existing ocular surface diseases, or systemic immunodeficiency [11]. Clinically, patients with infectious keratitis may present with a range of symptoms, including ocular pain, redness, photophobia, decreased vision, and discharge. A thorough ophthalmic examination using a slit-lamp microscope may reveal an epithelial defect, focal infiltrate, stromal edema, and, in some cases, an overlying hypopyon [12].

The management of IK must be aggressive and tailored to the type of pathogen suspected. Bacterial keratitis, often caused by *Staphylococcus*, *Streptococcus*, and *Pseudomonas* species, is typically treated with broad-spectrum topical antibiotics, which are later refined based on microbial culture and sensitivity results [9]. Viral keratitis, predominantly due to the *herpes simplex virus*, requires antiviral therapy [13]. Fungal keratitis, caused by organisms such as *Fusarium* or *Aspergillus*, is managed with topical antifungal agents [14]. Parasitic infections like *Acanthamoeba* keratitis, although less common, are particularly challenging to treat and necessitate the use of topical anti-amoebic medications [15].

Laboratory testing plays a pivotal role in diagnosing and managing infectious keratitis. Cultures from corneal scrapings can identify the causative organism and guide targeted therapy. Molecular techniques like polymerase chain reaction (PCR) offer rapid and sensitive detection of microbial DNA [16]. In vivo, confocal microscopy and anterior segment optical coherence tomography (ASOCT) are valuable non-invasive imaging modalities that can provide detailed visualization of the corneal layers and assist in diagnosing and monitoring treatment response [16].

The depth and severity of the infection also influence the choice of management strategy. For superficial keratitis, topical medications may suffice. However, fortified antibiotics or combination therapy may be necessary for deeper infections. In cases where there is no response to medical therapy or in the presence of complications such as impending perforation, surgical intervention becomes essential.

Surgical options include corneal debridement, therapeutic keratoplasty, and, in severe cases, corneal transplantation [17].

Preventive strategies are equally important in the management of infectious keratitis. These include patient education on contact lens care, avoidance of contact lens wear in high-risk environments such as swimming, and immediate evaluation of any ocular trauma. Public health measures, including improved access to clean water and sanitation, are critical in reducing the incidence of infectious keratitis in susceptible populations [18].

Overall, infectious keratitis requires a coordinated approach to management, encompassing accurate diagnosis, prompt initiation of therapy, and regular follow-up to monitor treatment efficacy and detect any complications. Advances in diagnostic technology and antimicrobial therapy continue to improve the prognosis for patients with infectious keratitis, but challenges remain, particularly in resource-limited settings where the disease burden is highest [19].

2 Pathophysiology

Infectious keratitis is a pathophysiological process where the cornea becomes inflamed due to an infection. This condition is initiated when pathogens such as bacteria, viruses, fungi, or parasites breach the protective barriers of the eye, often through a disruption in the corneal epithelium [11]. This disruption can occur due to factors like contact lens wear, eye trauma, or compromised immune defense. Once the pathogen invades the stromal tissue of the cornea, it triggers an inflammatory response [20]. This response involves the activation of the immune system, leading to an influx of inflammatory cells and mediators into the cornea. These cells work to eliminate the pathogen but can also cause collateral damage to corneal tissues. The resulting inflammation and tissue damage manifest as the symptoms of keratitis—pain, redness, blurred vision, and sensitivity to light. The host's immune system responds to this invasion with an inflammatory response aimed at eliminating the pathogen. This response includes the activation of innate immune cells, like neutrophils and macrophages, and the release of cytokines and chemokines, which help in fighting the infection but can also contribute to corneal damage [12].

In some cases, an excessive or prolonged immune response can lead to further corneal injury and scarring, exacerbating the severity of the disease. The balance between the virulence of the pathogen and the effectiveness of the host's immune response ultimately determines the progression and severity of infectious keratitis [21]. Effective management of the condition thus requires not only targeting the pathogen with appropriate antimicrobial therapy but also managing the inflammatory response to prevent excessive tissue damage. In severe cases, the infection and the associated immune response can lead to corneal ulceration, scarring, and even perforation, potentially causing significant vision impairment or loss. The specific pathophysiological mechanisms can vary based on the type of pathogen involved. For instance, bacterial infections often result in rapid, acute inflammation, whereas fungal infections might lead to more chronic and indolent processes. The severity and progression of infectious keratitis are influenced by factors such as the pathogen's virulence, the host's immune status, and the treatment's timeliness and effectiveness [19].

3 Clinical Presentation

Infectious keratitis is a serious eye infection that affects the cornea, often caused by bacteria, viruses, fungi, or parasites. The symptoms of infectious keratitis can vary depending on the underlying cause but generally include severe eye pain, redness, and irritation [2]. Patients may also experience blurred vision or sensitivity to light (photophobia) as the infection progresses. It is common for the affected eye to produce excessive tears or a thick, sticky discharge. The cornea may appear cloudy or have visible white spots in more advanced cases, indicating an ulcer or severe infection [22]. These symptoms can reduce vision quality and, if left untreated, might result in permanent vision loss. Early detection and treatment are crucial to prevent complications. If any of these symptoms are present, especially following an eye injury or contact lens use, seeking immediate medical attention is advised [9].

Differentiating between bacterial, viral, fungal, acanthamoeba, and Pythium keratitis is crucial for effective treatment, as the signs and symptoms vary between these infections. Bacterial keratitis typically presents with a rapid onset of pain, redness, and discharge, with the cornea showing a dense, central, white infiltrate that may develop into an ulcer (Fig. 1). Staphylococcus and Pseudomonas are common culprits, and they often cause a 'hypopyon,' a visible layer of white blood cells in the anterior chamber of the eye [9].

Viral keratitis, often caused by the herpes simplex virus, may start with a less aggressive presentation, including redness, tearing, and blurred vision. The key sign is a dendritic ulcer, which can be seen on corneal staining with fluorescein and presents as branching lesions on the cornea (Fig. 2) [23].

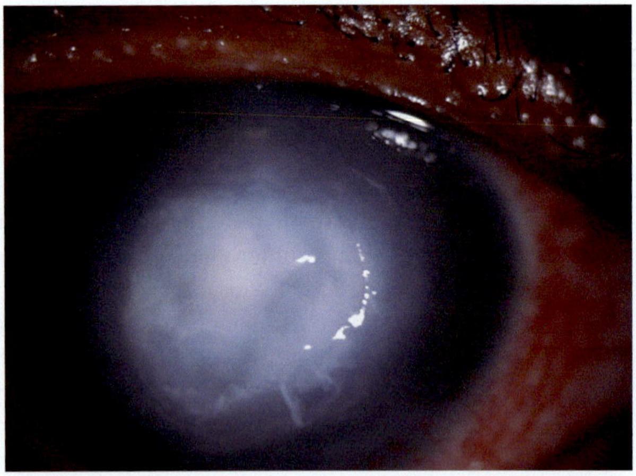

Fig. 1 Diffuse slit-lamp image of a patient with Pseudomonas keratitis depicting a full-thickness corneal infiltrate with a stromal melt

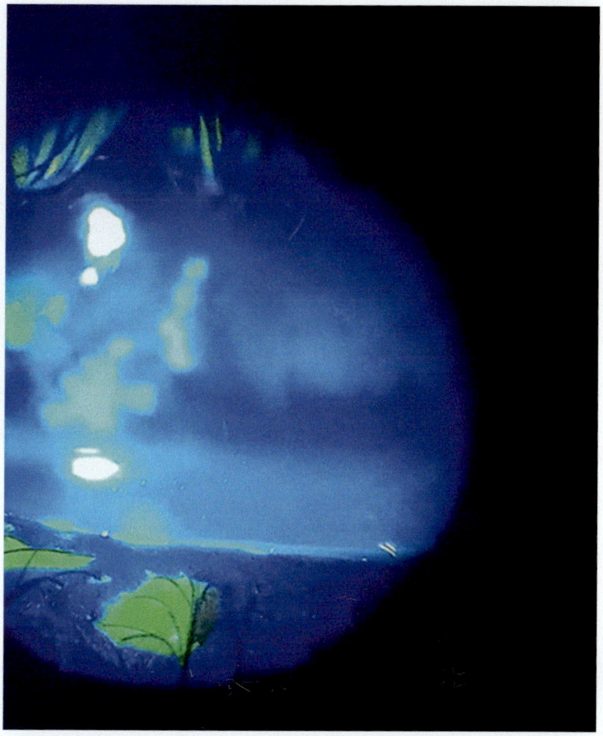

Fig. 2 Diffuse slit-lamp cobalt blue illumination image of a patient depicting multiple dendrites in a case of herpes simplex keratitis

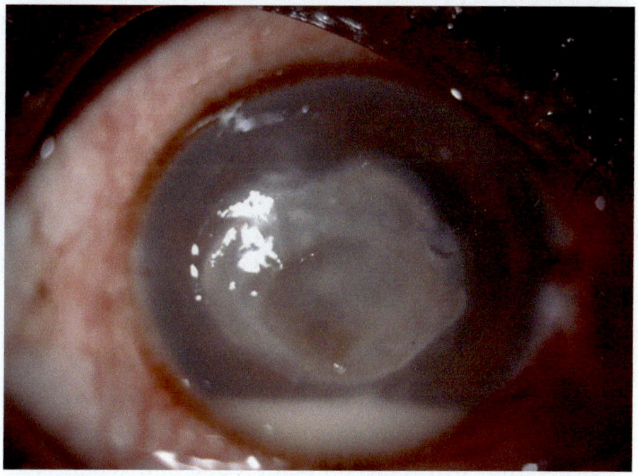

Fig. 3 Diffuse slit image of a patient with Curvularia keratitis depicting healing pigmented corneal infiltrate with hypopyon

Fungal keratitis, which can be due to various fungi like Fusarium or Aspergillus, typically has a slower onset. It presents with a grayish, feathery infiltrate and may include satellite lesions—small, separate opacities that surround the main infiltration. Patients may also experience a more significant sensation of a foreign body in the eye [21]. Hypopyon is usually immobile and maybe convex (Fig. 3).

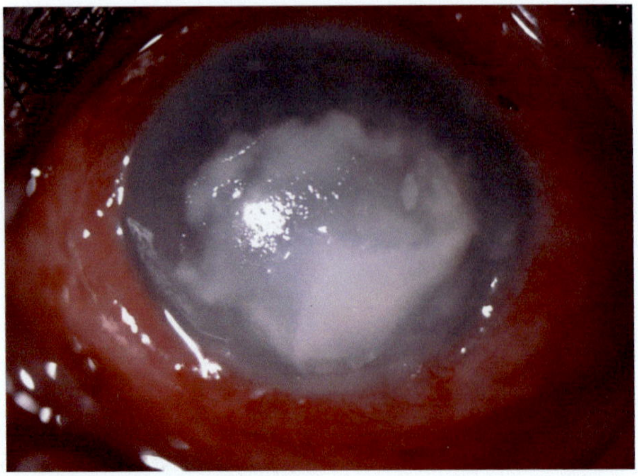

Fig. 4 Diffuse slit image of a patient with Pythium keratitis depicting cotton wool-like fluffy full-thickness corneal infiltrate with rapid inferior limbal spread 5 days post-trauma with vegetative matter

Acanthamoeba keratitis is often associated with contact lens wear, especially when exposed to contaminated water. Symptoms may mimic bacterial or viral keratitis initially but persist despite treatment. A key distinguishing feature is severe pain out of proportion to clinical findings. Ring-shaped stromal infiltrates may eventually appear [18].

Pythium keratitis, a rarer condition, resembles fungal keratitis but tends to be more aggressive. It features rapidly progressive ulcers and may show a tentacular projects, peripheral furrowing and early limbal spread with guttering, which is quite distinctive (Fig. 4). It is more prevalent in tropical regions and often requires aggressive treatment [24, 25]. In all cases, specialized laboratory tests are required for an accurate diagnosis, and an eye care professional should evaluate any of these signs promptly to avoid complications and loss of vision.

4 Diagnostic Approach

The diagnostic approach for IK is multifaceted, with an emphasis on the importance of accurate and timely diagnosis to prevent complications such as vision loss or corneal scarring. The process typically involves:

- **Clinical Examination**
  Initial assessment includes a patient history to identify risk factors such as contact lens use, recent eye trauma, or exposure to contaminated water. Symptom evaluation will focus on pain, redness, discharge, and visual changes [26].
- **Slit-Lamp Biomicroscopy**
  This is a critical tool in the evaluation of keratitis. A slit lamp allows for a detailed examination of the cornea, conjunctiva, and anterior chamber. It helps to identify the location and depth of the corneal lesion, epithelial defect, depth and extent of

infiltrate, endothelial plaques, and anterior chamber reactions, including hypopyon [27].

- **Fluorescein Staining Patterns**
  The application of fluorescein dye during slit-lamp examination can reveal distinct patterns. For example, dendritic ulcers are indicative of herpes simplex virus keratitis, whereas diffuse staining might suggest a more widespread epithelial breakdown, as seen in bacterial or fungal infections [28]. The staining is useful to locate the epithelial defect, check for seidels test in case of a perforation and also to assess the healing of epithelial defect.
- **Sample Collection**
  Optimal specimen acquisition is pivotal and must occur during the initial clinical evaluation before the commencement of antimicrobial treatment. Empirical therapy may be instituted contingent upon the outcomes of the smear analysis. The following are the specimens pertinent to the etiological determination of corneal ulcerations [29]:
- **Eyelid Swab**: Generally yields limited diagnostic utility.
- **Conjunctival Swab**: Typically of marginal diagnostic value.
- **Corneal Scraping**: This is the paramount specimen for diagnostic assessment, providing critical microbiological insights.
- **Contact Lens**: The procurement of the contact lens, its storage case, and the solution are mandatory for individuals who use contact lenses, as they can be a repository of pathogens [18].
- **Anterior Chamber Paracentesis (Hypopyon Aspirate):** This procedure is reserved for cases with profound ulceration or when there is an insufficient sample from corneal scraping to conduct an adequate analysis.

4.1 Laboratory Diagnosis

4.1.1 Corneal Scraping and Smear Analysis

The foundational approach for identifying corneal ulcers involves scrutinizing corneal scrapings and culturing tissue from the cornea. The Gram stain method is effective for bacterial infections, yielding 60–75% identification rates. For fungal infections, its effectiveness is noted to be between 35% and 50%. The use of a potassium hydroxide (KOH) preparation is recognized for its 76.3% sensitivity rate in pinpointing fungal keratitis. When dealing with fungal, Acanthamoeba, and Microsporidial keratitis, Calcofluor white stain proves to be beneficial. Standard culture media for bacterial growth include blood and chocolate agar. For fungal growth, media such as Sabouraud's dextrose agar or potato dextrose agar are preferred.

Meanwhile, acanthamoeba is typically cultivated on a non-nutrient agar that has been supplemented with Escherichia coli. In cases of fungal keratitis that do not respond to standard treatments, it is advisable to consider the possibility of *Pythium insidiosum* infection. The hyphae of this organism typically show a positive reaction to stains such as calcofluor-KOH, acridine orange hydrochloride, potassium

Table 1 Jones criteria for a confirmed positive culture in infectious keratitis

1	Clinical signs of infection and the cultivation of bacteria amounting to a count of 10 or greater colonies on a single solid medium and bacterial presence on a secondary medium
2	Recovery of an organism, with any level of growth observable, on two separate solid media
3	Identification of an organism in a single medium, supported by a positive result from a smear test
4	Should initial culture results return negative, there is a protocol to pause antibiotic therapy for a 24-h interval. After this hiatus, a new corneal scraping should be performed. Subsequently, samples are recultured and revaluated

iodide-sulphuric acid, and lactophenol blue. The Tzanck smear is a cytological diagnostic test that has been traditionally used to detect herpes simplex virus (HSV) infections, which are a common cause of ocular viral keratitis. Under microscopic examination, a positive Tzanck smear would show multinucleated giant cells and epithelial cells with characteristic cytopathic effects, such as ballooning degeneration. These findings can suggest a herpesvirus infection.

4.1.2 Culture Techniques

Samples from corneal scrapings are cultured on different media to isolate bacteria, fungi, or amoeba. Blood agar (aerobic bacteria, facultative anaerobic bacteria, fungi), chocolate agar (aerobic bacteria, facultative anaerobic bacteria, *Neisseria, Haemophilus, Moraxella*), Thioglycolate broth (aerobic bacteria, anaerobic bacteria), Sabouraud's dextrose agar (Fungi, Nocardia), brain heart infusion broth plate with antibiotic (Fungi, *Nocardia*), Cooked meat broth (anaerobic bacteria), Thayer martin blood agar plate (*Neisseria* species), Lowenstein–Jensen media (*Mycobacteria* species), Middlebrook-Cohn agar (*Mycobacteria species, Nocardia*), and non-nutrient agar with *E.* coli overlay for Acanthamoeba are commonly used. Jones criteria for confirmed positive culture cases in IK are given in Table 1.

4.1.3 Corneal Biopsy in Infectious Keratitis

A corneal biopsy may become necessary when infectious keratitis is strongly suspected, yet there is an absence of positive findings after two consecutive smear analyses and culture attempts. This step is considered especially when no discernible clinical response to initial empirical broad-spectrum antibiotic treatment exists. Additionally, corneal biopsy is advised for specific conditions, such as extensive fungal keratitis and stromal abscesses where the infection is situated deep within the corneal tissue.

4.2 Procedure for Corneal Biopsy

The biopsy procedure typically involves partial-thickness trephination using an appropriately sized trephine. This ensures the collection of a sufficient sample for diagnostic analysis. During the procedure, it is critical to steer clear of the visual axis to the greatest extent possible. A biopsy may be performed beneath a lamellar flap for lesions situated mid-stromal, such as those seen in infectious crystalline keratopathy, or for deeper stromal infections like fungal keratitis. This approach helps in obtaining a sample from the precise depth of the lesion.

4.2.1 Anterior Chamber Paracentesis

Anterior chamber paracentesis is an infrequently required diagnostic measure in the assessment of corneal ulcers. Nevertheless, it may be warranted in cases where there is a high clinical suspicion of keratomycosis but where corneal scrapings and biopsies have not yielded positive results. This procedure is particularly considered when there is observed advancement in corneal damage and when there is the presence or exacerbation of a hypopyon [30].

4.2.2 Molecular Diagnostics (PCR)

Polymerase chain reaction (PCR) testing can rapidly detect microbial DNA or RNA from small samples, offering a more sensitive and faster diagnosis, particularly for viral keratitis and atypical pathogens like Acanthamoeba or Pythium insidiosum [31].

4.2.3 In Vivo Confocal Microscopy

This non-invasive in vivo imaging technique provides high-resolution images of the cornea. It is beneficial for diagnosing fungal and acanthamoeba keratitis as it can visualize the characteristic structures like hyphae or double-walled cysts within the corneal stroma. The latest advancements in In Vivo Confocal Microscopy (IVCM) technology can aid in the early commencement of antifungal treatments and provide valuable insights into the patient's response to the therapy. Additionally, IVCM is emerging as a preferred diagnostic tool due to its non-invasive nature, speed, and high sensitivity. IVCM excels in detecting sizable and deeply embedded organisms that conventional corneal scraping might miss, such as filamentous fungi, Acanthamoeba, and Nocardia [32].

4.2.4 Anterior Segment Optical Coherence Tomography (ASOCT)

Techniques like ASOCT can provide detailed cross-sectional images of the cornea and are useful for assessing the depth of corneal infiltrates and ulcers. Furthermore, ASOCT is increasingly utilized for quantifying the extent of corneal infiltrates or scarring and tracking corneal thinning throughout treatment. This imaging provides an objective assessment that can be invaluable for managing the condition effectively [33].

4.2.5 Contemporary Approaches

The imperative for swift diagnostic capabilities has fostered enhancements to traditional methodologies and the emergence of novel techniques, including immunohistochemistry, fluorescence microscopy, enzyme-linked immunoassays, radioimmunoassay, and advanced molecular biology techniques like PCR. These cutting-edge methods have significantly reduced the diagnostic timeline for most ocular infections, with results now achievable within a span of 1–6 h [34].

4.2.6 Genomic Sequencing

Sequencing of the internal transcribed spacer (ITS) region of the fungal genome is a technique that significantly hastens the diagnosis of fungal keratitis, particularly in stubborn cases. This method's efficacy is well-documented in the identification of *Pythium* and other molds that do not form spores. Moreover, this molecular approach facilitates the identification of uncommon fungal pathogens. Examples include *Beauveria bassiana*, noted for its formidable resistance to antifungal medications, as well as *Colletotrichum gloeosporioides* and *Trametes betulina*. Each diagnostic tool has its strengths and may be used in conjunction with others to confirm the type of IK. Early and accurate diagnosis is essential to guide appropriate and effective treatment, reduce the risk of complications, and improve the outcomes for the patient. It is imperative that these diagnostic steps are performed promptly and interpreted by an eye care professional experienced in managing corneal diseases [35].

5 Differential Diagnosis

The differential diagnosis of infectious keratitis is crucial to ensure proper management and treatment. Here is a detailed approach:

5.1 Distinguishing Infectious from Non-infectious Keratitis

Infectious keratitis typically presents with pain, photophobia, reduced vision, and signs of infection like corneal infiltrates, edema, and ulceration. Non-infectious keratitis may have similar symptoms but often lacks purulent discharge or marked anterior chamber reaction. A history of trauma, contact lens wear, or prior ocular surgery may suggest an infectious etiology, whereas autoimmune conditions or dry eye syndrome might point toward non-infectious causes [36].

5.2 Other Causes of Red-Eye

- **Conjunctivitis:** Can be viral, bacterial, or allergic. It usually presents with diffuse redness, itching, and a watery or mucopurulent discharge, but the cornea is typically clear.
- **Episcleritis:** Involves inflammation of the episclera, causing localized or diffuse redness with minimal pain and no discharge.
- Scleritis: More severe, deep-seated eye redness and pain, often associated with systemic autoimmune diseases.
- **Acute Glaucoma:** Can mimic infectious keratitis but is distinguished by a mid-dilated pupil, high intraocular pressure, and a history of halos around lights [2].

5.3 Corneal Dystrophies and Degenerations Mimicking Infection

- **Corneal Dystrophies:** Genetic conditions such as Fuchs' endothelial dystrophy or lattice dystrophy might present with corneal changes, including haze and deposits, which can be confused with infection.
- **Corneal Degenerations:** Conditions like band keratopathy and Salzmann's nodular degeneration can cause corneal opacities and surface irregularity that may resemble infectious keratitis [1].

5.3.1 Management Strategies

The management of infectious keratitis involves a combination of medical and, if necessary, surgical strategies. Here is an outline of the various management approaches:

6 General Management Principles

Immediate commencement of treatment is critical to prevent corneal scarring or perforation.

Adjust therapy based on clinical response and laboratory results. Frequent monitoring of the corneal lesion is necessary. In severe cases, hospitalization may be required for close observation and intensive care [12].

6.1 Medical Management

6.1.1 Antibacterial Therapy

- **Empiric Therapy:** Broad-spectrum topical antibiotics like fluoroquinolones are often initiated while awaiting culture results.
- **Culture-Directed**: Once pathogens are identified, more specific antibiotics are chosen based on sensitivity patterns.

Bacterial Keratitis

It is a critical ocular condition that must be treated promptly due to its potential for rapid progression and severe complications. Immediate initiation of empirical antibiotic therapy is essential. This often involves a combination regimen covering a broad spectrum of Gram-positive and Gram-negative organisms. The standard treatment protocol typically includes:

- A fortified antibiotic solution such as cefazolin at 5% or 10% concentration combined with tobramycin at 1.3%.
- A fluoroquinolone such as moxifloxacin 0.5% or gatifloxacin 0.3% is also used in conjunction with tobramycin 1.3% [9].

When comparing fluoroquinolones with fortified eye drops, several factors are considered:

- **Cost:** Fluoroquinolones are generally less expensive than fortified drops.
- **Availability:** Fluoroquinolones are readily available, whereas fortified drops must be specially prepared.
- **Stability:** Fluoroquinolones are stable at room temperature, whereas fortified drops often require refrigeration to maintain potency.
- **Shelf Life:** Fluoroquinolones typically have a shelf life of up to 1 month, compared to 1 week for fortified drops.
- **Toxicity:** Fortified drops are generally more toxic than fluoroquinolones.
- **Efficacy:** Older generations of fluoroquinolones may have poor coverage against Gram-positive organisms, whereas fortified drops tend to have better coverage overall.

In clinical practice, the choice between fluoroquinolones and fortified antibiotics is made based on the severity of the infection, bacterial culture results, patient tolerance, and the potential for toxicity. Regular monitoring and adjustments to therapy may be required to ensure the best outcome for the patient [9].

The dosing frequency of eye drops is typically dictated by the severity of the condition. Standard practice involves initiating treatment with half-hourly administrations around the clock for the majority of patients. In cases of severe corneal ulcers, an initial loading dose may be employed, consisting of drops every 5 min for the first half-hour. The dosing intervals are then adjusted according to the clinical improvement observed [11]. For fortified drops, aminoglycosides such as gentamicin and tobramycin are utilized, providing robust coverage against gram-negative bacteria and efficacy against certain strains of staphylococci and streptococci, although they are less effective against pneumococci. Cefazolin is the cephalosporin most frequently employed in fortified drops, offering substantial activity against gram-positive bacteria that do not produce penicillinase.

Symptom management may include ancillary treatments such as cycloplegic medications, anti-glaucoma agents, artificial tears, and potentially topical corticosteroids.

Systemic antibiotics are considered in bacterial keratitis under specific circumstances such as:

- Corneal ulcers with actual or imminent perforation.
- Post-traumatic perforations.
- Involvement of the sclera.
- Development of endophthalmitis.
- Infections are caused by highly virulent pathogens like *Neisseria* and *Haemophilus*.

The Steroid for Corneal Ulcer Trial (SCUT) did not demonstrate a significant difference in the best-corrected visual acuity at 3 months between patients treated with topical corticosteroids versus placebo as an adjunctive therapy in the management of bacterial corneal ulcers. Additionally, the use of corticosteroids did not show an increased risk of corneal perforation [9].

Viral Keratitis; Herpes Simplex Keratitis

Antiviral Therapy

Topical antivirals such as trifluridine or ganciclovir are standard. Oral antiviral medications like acyclovir, valacyclovir, or famciclovir can be used, particularly for deep stromal involvement or for prophylaxis against recurrence. Available antiviral agents for treatment include acyclovir at a 3% concentration in ointment form, vidarabine also at 3%, trifluorothymidine at 1%, and idoxuridine at 1% [23]. It is crucial to reassess the condition if ulceration remains active beyond a 14-day treatment period. This evaluation is necessary to differentiate between a neurotrophic ulcer and ongoing infectious epithelial keratitis. A neurotrophic ulcer typically presents with smooth margins, in contrast to the irregular, scalloped edges often seen in infectious epithelial keratitis. In cases where infectious epithelial keratitis is ongoing, the possibility of antiviral resistance should be considered. Under these circumstances, initiating an alternative antiviral therapy may be warranted [13].

Fungal Keratitis

Antifungal Agents

Agents like natamycin, amphotericin B, or voriconazole are used depending on the type of fungus. Treatment duration is typically longer than for bacterial infections.

The principal categories of antifungal agents encompass:

- **Polyenes:** This class includes Natamycin, Nystatin, and Amphotericin B.
- **Azoles:** This group features Fluconazole, Itraconazole, Voriconazole, Posaconazole, and Ravuconazole.
- **Fluorinated Pyrimidines**, such as Flucytosine.
- **Echinocandins:** Including Caspofungin and Micafungin.

The typical treatment regimen for fungal infections follows a stepwise approach:

Topical Antifungals: The preferred choice is 5% Natamycin, administered every hour during the day and every 2 h at night. Based on the clinical response, the frequency is gradually reduced after 4–7 days [14].

Surface Debridement: This procedure aims to eliminate slough and reduce the infection load. Though its benefits are debated, it is still widely used by clinicians.

Adjustments for Worsening Conditions: If there is no improvement after 14 days, options include adding 0.15% Amphotericin B drops or 1% Voriconazole and revisiting the culture report.

Duration of Therapy: Treatment typically spans 3–4 weeks, with complete resolution often taking 4–8 weeks [21].

Antifungals, unlike antibacterials, have limitations such as reduced ocular penetration, limited bioavailability, potential epithelial toxicity, and availability issues.

Indications for systemic antifungals in fungal keratitis include:

- Perforated or imminent perforation of the corneal ulcer.
- Severe, deep ulcers involving more than two-thirds of the stromal depth.
- Large ulcers exceeding 6 mm in diameter.
- Cases following penetrating keratoplasty.
- Scleral involvement.
- Endophthalmitis.

Common systemic antifungals include Ketoconazole (200 mg twice daily), Fluconazole (200 mg twice daily), Itraconazole (100 mg twice daily), and Voriconazole (200 mg twice daily). Monitoring for adverse effects is crucial, including regular blood glucose, blood pressure, and liver function checks [22].

6.1.2 Targeted Drug Delivery

For approximately 20% of fungal ulcers resistant to medical therapy, targeted drug delivery is a viable option before considering surgery. This method ensures that the drug is delivered directly to the affected area. Techniques include intracameral, intracorneal, or intrastromal drug delivery. The agents used in these methods are Amphotericin B (5–7.5 μg per 0.1 mL in 5% dextrose) and Voriconazole (50–100 μg per 0.1 mL) [29].

Acanthamoeba Keratitis

Anti-amoebic Drugs

Combination therapy, including topical chlorhexidine, polyhexamethylene biguanide (PHMB), and propamidine isethionate, is effective. Oral agents like itraconazole or miltefosine may be added for severe cases.

The treatment of Acanthamoeba keratitis is challenging and often involves a combination of medications:

- **Biguanides:** The primary agents used are PHMB and chlorhexidine. These agents are effective against both the cystic and trophozoite forms of Acanthamoeba.
- **Aminoglycosides:** Drugs like neomycin may be used in combination with biguanides due to their efficacy against the trophozoite form [15].
- **Azole Antifungals:** Ketoconazole, fluconazole, or voriconazole can be effective due to their anti-acanthamoeba properties.
- **Propamidine Isethionate and Hexamidine:** These are effective against the trophozoite form and can be used as adjunctive therapy.
- **Topical Steroids:** The use of steroids is controversial and typically avoided in the initial phase due to the potential exacerbation of the infection. Steroids may be considered in later stages to control inflammation after infection control.
- **Pain Management:** Cycloplegics can be used for pain relief and to manage photophobia. Oral analgesics may also be necessary.

- **Debridement of Infected Tissue:** In some cases, removal of the infected corneal epithelium can enhance drug penetration [18].

Pythium Insidiosum Keratitis

Antifungal Drug

Historically, Pythium Insidiosum Keratitis (PIK) was treated with antifungals such as 5% Natamycin, 1% Voriconazole, 1% Itraconazole, and 2% Ketoconazole under the assumption that they were typical fungal ulcers. However, further understanding of Pythium's unique cell wall structure, which lacks ergosterol, has revealed the limited efficacy of these antifungals against it. Studies by Bagga et al. have shown that antibacterials are more effective than antifungals for PIK, indicating them as the preferred first-line treatment. Even though Gurnani et al. recognized some role for antifungals in PIK, particularly in initial treatments before culture confirmations, their success is limited. In cases presenting clinical features suggestive of fungal keratitis but with negative cultures for Pythium, antifungals are recommended until fungal keratitis is ruled out. Caspofungin, an inhibitor of beta-glucan synthase, shows some effectiveness against PIK but with transient results [37].

Antibacterial Drug Therapy

In vitro studies and rabbit models have indicated the efficacy of 0.2% Linezolid and 1% Azithromycin as first-line antibacterials for PIK. These drugs demonstrate superior effectiveness compared to antifungals. Linezolid, prepared from IV formulations or crushed capsules, and Azithromycin, either as an eye ointment or oral medication, have been used with a high degree of success. Monitoring for clinical improvement, such as reduction in ulcer size and inflammation, is crucial. Combination therapy with Linezolid and Azithromycin is recommended for larger, vision-affecting ulcers. Other effective antibiotics include tetracyclines, lincosamides, and oxazolidinones, among others [38].

Adjuvant Therapy in PIK Treatment

- **Anti-glaucoma Medications**: Beta-blockers and adrenergic agonists are used to manage secondary glaucoma or hypopyon, reducing intraocular pressure and alleviating pain.
- **Cycloplegic Medications**: Agents like atropine and cyclopentolate relieve pain from ciliary muscle spasms and prevent complications like synechiae formation.
- **Anti-inflammatory Medications**: In PIK and post-keratoplasty cases, oral anti-inflammatory drugs such as diclofenac and ibuprofen are crucial for managing inflammation and pain.

In summary, the treatment of PIK has evolved with a greater emphasis on antibacterials over antifungals, supported by recent research. Adjuvant therapies play a significant role in managing symptoms and preventing complications. Regular monitoring and adjustments based on clinical response are key to successful treatment outcomes [24].

Surgical Management

Indications for Surgical Intervention

- Unresponsive to medical therapy.
- Progressive corneal thinning or perforation.
- Significant visual axis opacification after the resolution of infection.

Procedures

- **Debridement:** Removal of infected or necrotic tissue to promote healing.
- **Keratoplasty:** Corneal transplantation may be necessary for tectonic support or visual rehabilitation.
- **Amniotic Membrane Transplantation:** Used for promoting healing, reducing inflammation, and as a temporary patch for small perforations [39].

Surgical intervention in cases of infectious keratitis is considered under specific circumstances, such as impending or actual perforation and non-healing corneal ulcers, particularly when there is a high microbial load. The decision to proceed with surgery should be based on a thorough evaluation of the patient's clinical progress. Surgical options aim to reduce microbial burden and provide structural support to the eye, especially in cases where corneal integrity is compromised due to thinning or perforation. Various surgical techniques are available, including:

- **Epithelial Removal and Anterior Lamellar Keratectomy:** Useful in fungal keratitis, this procedure involves regular debridement to remove organisms and necrotic material, thus enhancing antifungal drug penetration. Anterior lamellar keratectomy targets the removal of dense fungal filaments from the cornea and can be combined with phototherapeutic keratectomy for anterior stromal infiltrates [40].
- **Conjunctival Flaps:** This method is beneficial for stabilizing the epithelial surface in cases of persistent epithelial defects or progressive ulceration, especially in viral keratitis. Gunderson's flap, covering the entire surface with conjunctival tissue, is used in advanced cases to preserve the integrity of the globe [40].
- **Tissue Adhesives:** Cyanoacrylate adhesives are used for supporting areas of corneal thinning and sealing perforations up to 2 mm in diameter. A bandage contact lens (BCL) is applied post-adhesive application, and the adhesive is maintained until it spontaneously loosens or further surgical intervention is necessary [39].
- **Patch Graft:** Techniques include Tenon's patch graft for peripheral ulcers, multi-layered amniotic membrane grafts for severe thinning or small perforations, and tectonic patch grafts for 3–5 mm perforations [39].
- **Therapeutic Penetrating Keratoplasty:** A full-thickness graft is indicated for larger perforations (>5 mm). Postoperative management includes continued antimicrobial treatment and cautious use of steroids in fungal keratitis. Smaller grafts tend to yield better outcomes [40].

- **Collagen Cross-linking (CXL):** CXL is effective in refractory cases due to its bactericidal activity and the increased resistance of crosslinked corneas to enzymatic degradation by pathogens. In all surgical procedures, thorough preoperative assessment and careful postoperative follow-up are crucial for optimal outcomes. The choice of surgery depends on the ulcer's size, location, and the patient's overall eye health. Surgery is particularly crucial when conservative treatments fail or in cases of severe infection where preserving ocular integrity is a priority. Regular follow-up and potential modification of the management plan are essential based on the clinical course of the disease. It is important to manage patient expectations regarding the healing process and visual recovery, as corneal healing can be prolonged, and vision improvement may be gradual. Multidisciplinary care involving an infectious disease specialist, a microbiologist, and a cornea specialist may be beneficial in complex cases [41].

7 Complications and Prognosis

Infectious keratitis, a serious eye infection affecting the cornea, can have various complications and a varied prognosis depending on several factors, including the cause of the infection, the patient's overall health, and the timeliness and effectiveness of treatment.

7.1 Complications of Infectious Keratitis

- **Corneal Scarring:** This is one of the most common complications. The infection can lead to scarring, which may cause permanent vision impairment or even blindness if the scar is centrally located.
- **Corneal Ulceration:** The infection can progress to create ulcers on the cornea. Deep ulcers can lead to corneal perforation, a severe condition that can result in vision loss.
- **Secondary Infections:** If the primary infection is not adequately treated, it can lead to secondary infections in the eye or other parts of the body.
- **Chronic Eye Pain:** Some patients experience ongoing eye pain, even after controlling the infection.
- **Hypopyon** is the accumulation of white blood cells in the anterior chamber of the eye, indicating a severe infection.
- **Spread of Infection:** In rare cases, the infection can spread to other parts of the eye, leading to conditions like endophthalmitis, which is an inflammation of the interior of the eye and can be sight-threatening [42].

7.2 Prognosis of Infectious Keratitis

The prognosis for infectious keratitis varies:

- **Early Diagnosis and Treatment:** If diagnosed and treated early, many patients recover completely without any permanent vision loss [11].
- **Type of Infectious Agent:** The causative organism affects the prognosis. Bacterial keratitis generally has a better prognosis than fungal or parasitic keratitis, which are often more challenging to treat [11, 12].
- **Underlying Health Conditions:** Patients with pre-existing eye conditions or systemic health issues, like diabetes or a compromised immune system, may have a poorer prognosis.
- **Adherence to Treatment:** The patient's adherence to treatment protocols, including the use of prescribed medications and follow-up appointments, significantly impacts the outcome.
- **Severity at Presentation:** More severe infections at the time of presentation tend to have a worse prognosis, particularly if the central cornea is involved or if there is a deep corneal ulcer.
- **Recurrence:** Some forms of keratitis, particularly those caused by herpes simplex virus, can recur, potentially worsening the long-term prognosis [11].

In conclusion, infectious keratitis can lead to serious complications, including vision loss, if not promptly and effectively treated. The prognosis varies widely based on the causative organism, the severity of the infection at diagnosis, the patient's overall health, and the effectiveness of treatment. Regular follow-up and adherence to treatment are crucial for a favorable outcome.

8 Prevention and Public Health Strategies

Preventing infectious keratitis involves several public health strategies and personal hygiene practices, particularly for individuals who wear contact lenses, are exposed to environmental risks, or have pre-existing ocular conditions [17]. Here is a detailed write-up on the prevention of infectious keratitis under the specified heads:

8.1 Contact Lens Hygiene

- **Proper Hand Washing:** Always wash hands with soap and water and dry them with a lint-free towel before handling contact lenses.
- **Disinfect Contact Lenses:** Use only the recommended type of disinfecting solution to clean and store contact lenses. Never use tap water, saliva, or non-sterile solutions [20].
- **Replace Lenses as Directed:** Follow the eye care professional's recommendations for replacement intervals for contact lenses and cases.
- **Avoid Sleeping in Contact Lenses:** Unless specifically designed for overnight wear, do not sleep in contact lenses to reduce the risk of infection [20].
- **Respect Water Exposure Guidelines**: Do not swim or shower while wearing contact lenses to prevent exposure to waterborne pathogens.

- **No Lens Sharing:** Never share contact lenses with others. This can spread microorganisms that may lead to infection.

8.2 Protective Eyewear

- **Use of Safety Glasses:** In environments with dust, chemicals, or potential for injury, protective eyewear should be used to prevent corneal abrasions, which can become infected.
- **Sports Eyewear:** Wear protective eyewear during sports to shield the eyes from injury and possible subsequent infection.
- **UV Protection**: Use sunglasses that block UV rays to protect the cornea and surrounding ocular tissues from UV damage, which can compromise the ocular surface [11].

8.3 Prompt Treatment of Ocular Surface Disease

- **Regular Eye Examinations:** Routine eye check-ups can help in the early detection and treatment of ocular surface diseases, preventing the progression to keratitis.
- **Manage Dry Eye**: Adequate treatment of dry eye syndrome is crucial as it can compromise the ocular surface and make it more susceptible to infections.
- **Treat Lid Margin Diseases:** Conditions such as blepharitis should be managed promptly to maintain a healthy ocular surface.
- **Control Inflammation:** The use of anti-inflammatory medications, as prescribed, can help control ocular surface inflammation and reduce the risk of infection [12].

8.4 Public Health Strategies

- **Education Campaigns:** Public health campaigns to educate about the risks associated with poor contact lens hygiene and the importance of protective eyewear.
- **Access to Eye Care Services:** Ensuring that communities have access to quality eye care services for promptly diagnosing and treating ocular surface diseases.
- **Surveillance Systems:** Establish surveillance systems to monitor the incidence of infectious keratitis and to identify outbreaks related to contact lens products or solutions.
- **Regulation of Contact Lens Solutions:** Ensuring that contact lens solutions on the market are safe and effective and recalling products associated with increased risk of infection.
- **Research and Development:** Supporting research into better materials for contact lenses and more effective antimicrobial contact lens solutions [2].

By implementing these strategies, it is possible to reduce the incidence of infectious keratitis significantly. Public health initiatives combined with individual practices can contribute to improved ocular health and decrease the burden of this potentially serious eye infection.

9 Recent Advances

Recent advances in the management of IK have shown promising developments across various aspects of treatment and prevention. Here is a detailed overview under the specified headings:

9.1 Novel Pharmacotherapeutics

- **Targeted Antimicrobial Therapy:** Advances in pharmacotherapeutics include the development of newer antimicrobial agents that are more specific to the causative organisms of keratitis. These agents aim to reduce the resistance seen with traditional antibiotics [24].
- **Antimicrobial Peptides:** Research is exploring the use of antimicrobial peptides as potential therapeutic agents due to their broad-spectrum activity and reduced likelihood of developing resistance [43].
- **Collagen Cross-Linking (CXL):** Though originally developed for keratoconus, CXL is being investigated for its ability to increase corneal rigidity and halt the progression of corneal melting in bacterial keratitis [41].
- **Drug Delivery Systems:** Improvements in drug delivery, such as contact lenses with embedded medications or slow-release corneal inserts, ensure that therapeutic levels of drugs are maintained over a longer period, improving efficacy [44].

9.2 Advances in Surgical Techniques

- **Phototherapeutic Keratectomy (PTK):** This laser surgery technique can be used to remove superficial corneal scars caused by keratitis and is increasingly precise with recent technological advancements [45].
- **Lamellar Keratoplasty**: Advancements in partial-thickness corneal transplants allow for the selective replacement of diseased corneal tissue while preserving healthy parts, resulting in better outcomes and reduced rejection rates [46].
- **Amniotic Membrane Transplantation:** This surgical technique is used more frequently in the treatment of persistent epithelial defects and as a biological bandage after debridement for infectious keratitis [47].

9.3 Biomarkers for Early Detection

- **Genetic Markers:** Research into genetic markers that may predispose individuals to certain types of keratitis could allow for earlier identification and targeted prevention strategies.
- **Tear Fluid Analysis:** The analysis of tear fluid for specific enzymes or inflammatory markers associated with infection can facilitate early detection and treatment [48].
- **In Vivo Confocal Microscopy:** This imaging technique allows for the non-invasive examination of the cornea at a cellular level, which can help in the early diagnosis of microbial keratitis before clinical signs become apparent [32].

9.4 Vaccination for Prevention of Viral Keratitis

- **Herpes Simplex Virus (HSV) Vaccine:** While still under development, there is ongoing research into vaccines for HSV, which is a common cause of viral keratitis. The aim is to reduce the incidence and severity of HSV-related ocular disease [49].
- **Adenovirus Vaccine:** Research is also being conducted into vaccines for adenovirus, which causes epidemic keratoconjunctivitis and can lead to keratitis [50].
- **Public Health Vaccination Programs:** The implementation of widespread vaccination programs could significantly reduce the incidence of viral keratitis, particularly in regions where it is endemic.

These recent advances represent a multifaceted approach to the management of infectious keratitis, focusing on improved treatment modalities, surgical interventions, early detection, and preventative measures. Continued research and development in these areas hold the promise of better outcomes for patients affected by this condition.

10 Future Directions

The future directions in managing and understanding infectious keratitis are driven by ongoing research and the evolving landscape of microbial resistance. Addressing research gaps, exploring the potential of gene therapy, and the need for new antibiotics are at the forefront of this field. Here is a detailed write-up on these aspects:

10.1 Research Gaps

- **Pathogen-Specific Data**: There is a need for more comprehensive data on the prevalence and virulence of specific pathogens in different geographic and

demographic populations. This information would help in developing targeted therapies.
- **Disease Mechanisms:** The exact mechanisms by which different pathogens affect the cornea and cause varying levels of damage are not fully understood. Research is needed to elucidate these processes at the molecular level.
- **Host Response:** A better understanding of the host immune response to corneal infections could lead to improved treatment strategies that minimize inflammation and scarring.
- **Long-Term Outcomes:** There is a scarcity of data on the long-term outcomes of infectious keratitis, particularly regarding visual acuity, recurrence rates, and quality of life.
- **Prevention Strategies:** Research into effective prevention strategies, especially in regions with high incidence rates, is needed to reduce the disease burden [51].

10.2 Potential for Gene Therapy

- **Genetic Vulnerabilities:** Identifying genetic factors that make individuals more susceptible to keratitis could lead to gene therapies that strengthen the cornea's defenses against infection.
- **Gene Editing:** Techniques like CRISPR/Cas9 offer the potential to edit genes that may be involved in the pathogenesis or progression of keratitis, possibly preventing the disease before it manifests.
- **Delivery Mechanisms:** Research into efficient and safe delivery methods for gene therapy to the cornea is ongoing. Viral vectors, nanoparticles, and mechanical methods like electroporation are being explored.
- **Regenerative Medicine:** Gene therapy might be used 1 day to promote corneal healing and regeneration, reducing the risk of scarring and vision loss following infection.

10.3 Development of Resistance and Need for New Antibiotics

- **Surveillance Programs:** Global surveillance programs are needed to monitor trends in antibiotic resistance among pathogens causing keratitis. This data can inform the development of new antibiotics.
- **Novel Antibiotics:** There is an urgent need to develop new antibiotics that work through different mechanisms to overcome resistance. Research is focused on finding compounds with unique targets in bacterial, fungal, and viral pathogens.
- **Antibiotic Stewardship:** Programs that promote the judicious use of antibiotics are essential to slow the development of resistance. Education for both healthcare providers and patients is a crucial component.
- **Alternative Therapies:** Exploring non-antibiotic therapies, such as bacteriophage therapy, antimicrobial peptides, and host-defense modulators, is crucial as resistance continues to grow.

10.4 Combination Therapies

Using combinations of antibiotics or other types of treatments may help overcome resistance and improve outcomes [52].

The future directions in the battle against infectious keratitis involve a multi-pronged approach that encompasses filling research gaps, harnessing the potential of gene therapy, and developing new antimicrobial agents to overcome resistance. These strategies require a global effort and collaboration across scientific disciplines to ensure that progress continues in preventing and treating this vision-threatening condition.

10.5 Importance of a Multidisciplinary Approach

A multidisciplinary approach is crucial in managing infectious keratitis effectively. This involves:

- **Ophthalmologists**: Leading the diagnosis and treatment efforts, including surgical interventions.
- **Microbiologists:** Providing expertise in identifying the causative pathogens and their sensitivity patterns.
- **Pharmacists:** Assisting with the optimal selection and dosing of antimicrobial agents.
- **Infectious Disease Specialists:** Offering guidance on systemic infections and complications.
- **Primary Care Physicians:** Participating in early recognition and referral, especially in community settings.
- **Public Health Professionals:** Implementing prevention strategies and surveillance for outbreaks.

Collaboration across these disciplines ensures comprehensive patient care, from initial presentation to long-term management, including the rehabilitation of vision if impairment occurs.

10.6 Call for Further Research

Despite advancements, significant challenges remain, and further research is essential:

- **Understanding Pathogen Behavior**: More research is needed to understand the evolving patterns of pathogen behavior, particularly in the context of climate change and global travel.
- **Host Immunity:** Investigating the host immune response to corneal infections could yield insights into new therapeutic targets.

- **Resistance Mechanisms:** Understanding how resistance develops and spreads among pathogens is critical to developing new antimicrobial strategies.
- **Gene Therapy and Regenerative Medicine:** Exploring the potential of gene therapy and stem cell-based regenerative medicine could offer novel treatment avenues.
- **Vaccines:** Research into vaccines for preventing viral keratitis, particularly for herpes simplex virus, requires ongoing investment and innovation.
- **Public Health Interventions:** Evaluating the effectiveness of public health interventions on the incidence and severity of infectious keratitis can guide future prevention efforts.
- **Global Health Disparities:** Addressing disparities in the incidence and outcomes of infectious keratitis across different regions is essential, necessitating research sensitive to diverse populations' needs [53].

11 Conclusion

Infectious keratitis remains a significant cause of ocular morbidity and potential visual loss worldwide. Our current understanding of infectious keratitis has expanded considerably, yet the condition continues to pose a threat to vision health. A unified, multidisciplinary approach coupled with an ongoing commitment to research is paramount to continue improving prevention, diagnosis, and treatment strategies, with the ultimate goal of preserving sight and improving patient outcomes.

12 Summary of Current Understanding

Infectious keratitis is an infection of the cornea caused by bacteria, viruses, fungi, or parasites. The severity of the infection can range from mild irritation to severe inflammation, leading to corneal scarring and vision impairment. Key factors in the pathogenesis of infectious keratitis include the pathogen's virulence, the integrity of the ocular surface, and the host immune response.

The standard of care involves prompt antimicrobial treatment, often guided by laboratory cultures and sensitivity testing. However, the rise of antimicrobial resistance has complicated treatment strategies. The introduction of newer pharmacotherapeutics, advancements in corneal transplantation, and the development of molecular diagnostic tools have improved outcomes for many patients [54].

References

1. Ting DSJ, Ho CS, Deshmukh R, Said DG, Dua HS. Infectious keratitis: an update on epidemiology, causative microorganisms, risk factors, and antimicrobial resistance. Eye (Lond). 2021;35(4):1084–101.

2. Cabrera-Aguas M, Khoo P, Watson SL. Infectious keratitis: a review. Clin Exp Ophthalmol. 2022;50(5):543–62.
3. Ung L, Bispo PJM, Shanbhag SS, Gilmore MS, Chodosh J. The persistent dilemma of microbial keratitis: global burden, diagnosis, and antimicrobial resistance. Surv Ophthalmol. 2019;64(3):255–71.
4. Erie JC, Nevitt MP, Hodge DO, Ballard DJ. Incidence of ulcerative keratitis in a defined population from 1950 through 1988. Arch Ophthalmol. 1993;111(12):1665–71.
5. Upadhyay MP, Karmacharya PC, Koirala S, Shah DN, Shakya S, Shrestha JK, Bajracharya H, Gurung CK, Whitcher JP. The Bhaktapur eye study: ocular trauma and antibiotic prophylaxis for the prevention of corneal ulceration in Nepal. Br J Ophthalmol. 2001;85(4):388–92.
6. Jeng BH, Gritz DC, Kumar AB, Holsclaw DS, Porco TC, Smith SD, Whitcher JP, Margolis TP, Wong IG. Epidemiology of ulcerative keratitis in Northern California. Arch Ophthalmol. 2010;128(8):1022–8.
7. Green M, Carnt N, Apel A, Stapleton F. Queensland Microbial Keratitis Database: 2005–2015. Br J Ophthalmol. 2019;103(10):1481–6.
8. Gonzales CA, Srinivasan M, Whitcher JP, Smolin G. Incidence of corneal ulceration in Madurai district, South India. Ophthalmic Epidemiol. 1996;3(3):159–66.
9. Al-Mujaini A, Al-Kharusi N, Thakral A, Wali UK. Bacterial keratitis: perspective on epidemiology, clinico-pathogenesis, diagnosis and treatment. Sultan Qaboos Univ Med J. 2009;9(2):184–95.
10. Lin TY, Yeh LK, Ma DH, Chen PY, Lin HC, Sun CC, Tan HY, Chen HC, Chen SY, Hsiao CH. Risk factors and microbiological features of patients hospitalized for microbial keratitis: a 10-year study in a referral center in Taiwan. Medicine (Baltimore). 2015;94(43):e1905.
11. Gurnani B, Kaur K. Bacterial keratitis. In: StatPearls [Internet]. Treasure Island: StatPearls Publishing; 2023. PMID: 34662023.
12. Singh P, Gupta A, Tripathy K. Keratitis. In: StatPearls [Internet]. Treasure Island: StatPearls Publishing; 2023. PMID: 32644440.
13. Labib BA, Chigbu DI. Clinical management of herpes simplex virus keratitis. Diagnostics. 2022;12(10):2368.
14. Atta S, Perera C, Kowalski RP, Jhanji V. Fungal keratitis: clinical features, risk factors, treatment, and outcomes. J Fungi. 2022;8(9):962.
15. Varacalli G, Di Zazzo A, Mori T, Dohlman TH, Spelta S, Coassin M, Bonini S. Challenges in acanthamoeba keratitis: a review. J Clin Med. 2021;10(5):942.
16. Gupta N, Tandon R. Investigative modalities in infectious keratitis. Indian J Ophthalmol. 2008;56(3):209–13.
17. Gokhale NS. Medical management approach to infectious keratitis. Indian J Ophthalmol. 2008;56(3):215–20.
18. Carnt N, Stapleton F. Strategies for the prevention of contact lens-related Acanthamoeba keratitis: a review. Ophthalmic Physiol Opt. 2016;36(2):77–92.
19. Austin A, Lietman T, Rose-Nussbaumer J. Update on the management of infectious keratitis. Ophthalmology. 2017;124(11):1678–89.
20. Fleiszig SMJ, Kroken AR, Nieto V, Grosser MR, Wan SJ, Metruccio MME, Evans DJ. Contact lens-related corneal infection: intrinsic resistance and its compromise. Prog Retin Eye Res. 2020;76:100804.
21. Wu J, Zhang WS, Zhao J, Zhou HY. Review of clinical and basic approaches of fungal keratitis. Int J Ophthalmol. 2016;9(11):1676–83.
22. Klotz SA, Penn CC, Negvesky GJ, Butrus SI. Fungal and parasitic infections of the eye. Clin Microbiol Rev. 2000;13(4):662–85.
23. Koganti R, Yadavalli T, Naqvi RA, Shukla D, Naqvi AR. Pathobiology and treatment of viral keratitis. Exp Eye Res. 2021;205:108483.
24. Gurnani B, Kaur K. Understanding barriers, recommended solutions, and future prospects for the diagnosis and management of Pythium insidiosum keratitis. Indian J Ophthalmol. 2023;71(12):3584–6.

25. Cao B, Gonugunta VT, Radhakrishnan N, Lalitha P, Gurnani B, Kaur K, Iyer G, Agarwal S, Srinivasan B, Keenan JD, Prajna NV. Outcomes of Pythium keratitis: a meta-analysis of individual patient data. Curr Ophthalmol Rep. 2022;10(4):198–208.
26. Ting DSJ, Gopal BP, Deshmukh R, Seitzman GD, Said DG, Dua HS. Diagnostic armamentarium of infectious keratitis: a comprehensive review. Ocul Surf. 2022;23:27–39.
27. Dahlgren MA, Lingappan A, Wilhelmus KR. The clinical diagnosis of microbial keratitis. Am J Ophthalmol. 2007;143(6):940–4.
28. Moshirfar M, Hopping GC, Vaidyanathan U, Liu H, Somani AN, Ronquillo YC, Hoopes PC. Biological staining and culturing in infectious keratitis: controversy in clinical utility. Med Hypothesis Discovery Innovation Ophthalmol. 2019;8(3):145–51.
29. Toumasis P, Tsantes AG, Tsiogka A, Samonis G, Vrioni G. From clinical suspicion to diagnosis: a review of diagnostic approaches and challenges in fungal keratitis. J Clin Med. 2024;13(1):286.
30. Sridhar MS, Sharma S, Gopinathan U, Rao GN. Anterior chamber tap: diagnostic and therapeutic indications in the management of ocular infections. Cornea. 2002;21(7):718–22.
31. Gurnani B, Kaur K. Predicting prognosis based on regional prevalence, ulcer morphology and treatment strategy in vision-threatening *Pythium insidiosum* keratitis. Clin Ophthalmol. 2023;17:1307–14.
32. Brasnu E, Bourcier T, Dupas B, Degorge S, Rodallec T, Laroche L, Borderie V, Baudouin C. In vivo confocal microscopy in fungal keratitis. Br J Ophthalmol. 2007;91(5):588–91.
33. Abdelghany AA, D'Oria F, Alio Del Barrio J, Alio JL. The value of anterior segment optical coherence tomography in different types of corneal infections: an update. J Clin Med. 2021;10(13):2841.
34. Gupta N, Varshney A, Ramappa M, Basu S, Romano V, Acharya M, Gaur A, Kapur N, Singh A, Shah G, Chaudhary I, Patel N, Tiwari A, Kate A, Sangwan V, Mathur U. Role of AS-OCT in managing corneal disorders. Diagnostics. 2022;12(4):918.
35. Agarwal S, Khan TA, Vanathi M, Srinivasan B, Iyer G, Tandon R. Update on diagnosis and management of refractory corneal infections. Indian J Ophthalmol. 2022;70(5):1475–90.
36. Srinivasan M, Mascarenhas J, Prashanth CN. Distinguishing infective versus noninfective keratitis. Indian J Ophthalmol. 2008;56(3):203–7.
37. Gurnani B, Christy J, Narayana S, Rajkumar P, Kaur K, Gubert J. Retrospective multifactorial analysis of *Pythium keratitis* and review of literature. Indian J Ophthalmol. 2021;69(5):1095–101.
38. Gurnani B, Kaur K, Kumar T. Commentary: current concepts, recent updates, and future treatment options for *Pythium insidiosum* keratitis. Indian J Ophthalmol. 2023;71(5):1874–6.
39. Said DG, Rallis KI, Al-Aqaba MA, Ting DSJ, Dua HS. Surgical management of infectious keratitis. Ocul Surf. 2023;28:401–12.
40. Upadhyay MP, Srinivasan M, Whitcher JP. Diagnosing and managing microbial keratitis. Community Eye Health. 2015;28(89):3–6.
41. Alio JL, Abbouda A, Valle DD, Del Castillo JM, Fernandez JA. Corneal cross linking and infectious keratitis: a systematic review with a meta-analysis of reported cases. J Ophthalmic Inflamm Infect. 2013;3(1):47.
42. Agrawal V. First aid for complications of infectious keratitis. Indian J Ophthalmol. 2008;56(3):221–2.
43. Mba IE, Nweze EI. Antimicrobial peptides therapy: an emerging alternative for treating drug-resistant bacteria. Yale J Biol Med. 2022;95(4):445–63.
44. Rykowska I, Nowak I, Nowak R. Soft contact lenses as drug delivery systems: a review. Molecules. 2021;26(18):5577.
45. Rathi VM, Vyas SP, Sangwan VS. Phototherapeutic keratectomy. Indian J Ophthalmol. 2012;60(1):5–14.
46. Espandar L, Carlson AN. Lamellar keratoplasty: a literature review. J Ophthalmol. 2013;2013:894319.

47. Dallal MMS, Nikkhahi F, Imeni SM, Molaei S, Hosseini SK, Kalafi Z, Yazdi SS, Mirzaei HMA. Amniotic membrane transplantation for persistent epithelial defects and ulceration due to *Pseudomonas* keratitis in a rabbit model. J Ophthalmic Vis Res. 2021;16(4):552–7.
48. Jung JH, Ji YW, Hwang HS, Oh JW, Kim HC, Lee HK, Kim KP. Proteomic analysis of human lacrimal and tear fluid in dry eye disease. Sci Rep. 2017;7(1):13363.
49. Krishnan R, Stuart PM. Developments in vaccination for herpes simplex virus. Front Microbiol. 2021;12:798927.
50. Gray GC, Erdman DD. Adenovirus Vaccines. Plotkin's Vaccines. 2018:121–133.e8. https://doi.org/10.1016/B978-0-323-35761-6.00010-9.
51. Ong ZZ, Sadek Y, Liu X, Qureshi R, Liu SH, Li T, Sounderajah V, Ashrafian H, Ting DSW, Said DG, Mehta JS, Burton MJ, Dua HS, Ting DSJ. Diagnostic performance of deep learning in infectious keratitis: a systematic review and meta-analysis protocol. BMJ Open. 2023;13(5):e065537.
52. Verma S, Singh A, Varshney A, Chandru RA, Acharya M, Rajput J, Sangwan VS, Tiwari AK, Bhowmick T, Tiwari A. Infectious keratitis: an update on role of epigenetics. Front Immunol. 2021;12:765890.
53. Ting DSJ, Chodosh J, Mehta JS. Achieving diagnostic excellence for infectious keratitis: a future roadmap. Front Microbiol. 2022;13:1020198.
54. Gurnani B, Kaur K, Venugopal A, Srinivasan B, Bagga B, Iyer G, Christy J, Prajna L, Vanathi M, Garg P, Narayana S, Agarwal S, Sahu S. *Pythium insidiosum* keratitis—a review. Indian J Ophthalmol. 2022;70(4):1107–20.

Advances in Glaucoma

Parul Ichhpujani and Shibal Bhartiya

1 Introduction

Glaucoma management is at the cusp of monumental change. While there are exciting possibilities emerging for its diagnosis, and therapeutic interventions, clinical scientists across the globe are looking increasingly at the quality of life of glaucoma patients. Research is being focused at not only genetics and gene therapy for glaucoma, but also at technologies that will enable better patient compliance with conventional anti glaucoma medications (AGMs); as well safer, and more effective surgical options [1, 2].

The clinical experience with respect to these technologies, expectedly, is limited, and so, their acceptability for both patients and glaucoma practitioners alike is a barrier for their early adoption. It is therefore imperative that a concerted effort be made towards education of patients and caregivers, as well as the health care team comprising of optometrists, general ophthalmologists, and glaucoma surgeons. It is only then that the patient will be able to benefit from the latest advances in glaucoma management. This chapter will cover the recent advances in glaucoma diagnostics, newer drugs as well as visual rehabilitation for glaucoma management.

P. Ichhpujani (✉)
Department of Ophthalmology, Government Medical College and Hospital, Chandigarh, India

S. Bhartiya
Department of Ophthalmology, Marengo Asis Hospitals, Gurugram, Haryana, India

D. Shu et al. (eds.), *Current Advances in Optometry*, Current Practices in Ophthalmology, https://doi.org/10.1007/978-981-97-8140-9_4

2 Glaucoma Diagnostics

Home Tonometry: Glaucoma treatment is currently based on a snapshot of an "in-office" intraocular pressure (IOP) measurement, twice or thrice a year. Recent literature has shown that the "at-home" tonometry can significantly alter IOP management. It allows measurement of diurnal fluctuations in IOP by providing a more holistic view of the IOP profile outside the clinic, which can help understand disease progression and therefore guide change in treatment strategy. The Icare Home (Icare Inc., USA) tonometer, which uses rebound tonometry, is easy to use as it does not require the administration of a topical anaesthetic. The patient needs to rest the instrument against his or her forehead and align the device in front of the cornea with the help of a light ring surrounding the probe. After correct positioning, when the ring turns green, a button needs to be pressed for the measurement. This tonometer records six consecutive IOP measurements and the average IOP along with the date and time of measurement are saved to a cloud database. However, nearly 10% of glaucoma patients are not able to operate this tonometer properly [3]. Nearly 9% of readings vary by more than 3 mm Hg from the gold standard, Goldmann applanation tonometry (GAT) and 2% of readings vary by more than 5 mm Hg [4]. A recent study has shown that patients can be taught to perform self-tonometry remotely using a remote video link [5].

Home tonometry can aid in the detection of IOP spikes, especially in patients with pigmentary or pseudoexfoliative glaucoma (PEXG), angle closure glaucoma (ACG) or in paediatric or postoperative patients.

A. ***Implantable sensors:*** The development of implantable sensors for continuous IOP monitoring has been possible due to the technological advances in the microelectromechanical systems (MEMS) and microfluidics. These sensors are being embedded in a contact lens or integrated into a tonometry device or embedded intraocularly [6]. Currently available continuous pressure monitoring systems include the EYEMATE® (Implandata Ophthalmic Products GmbH, Germany) and Triggerfish® (Sensimed AG, Switzerland). These are yet to be used routinely in clinical practice.

   Triggerfish Contact Lens Sensor (CLS): The SENSIMED Triggerfish is a soft silicone, contact lens with a circumferential sensor consisting of two platinum titanium strain gauges, which measure the changes in the radius of curvature of the cornea. The contact lens is available in three base curves sizes, 8.4, 8.7, and 9 mm. A wireless antenna adherent on the periocular surface receives an output signal transmitted by a microprocessor. The strain gauge takes 300 readings over a 30-s period every 5 min, giving 86,400 data points over a 24-h period (Fig. 1). Bluetooth connection allows this data to be transferred to a computer for analysis. The data points are measured in millivolt equivalents and are relative to the first reading (zero). The Triggerfish CLS does not give an estimate of absolute IOP.

   Eyemate-IO intraocular version: The Eyemate (Implandata; Hannover, Germany) is a new implantable device for continuous, long-term IOP monitor-

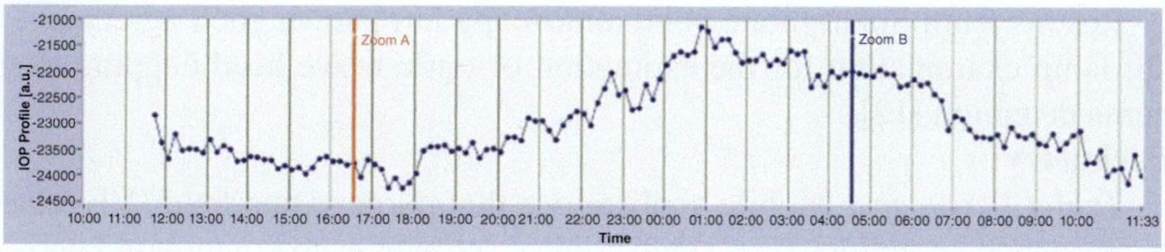

Fig. 1 A 24 h pressure profile obtained using Triggerfish

ing. It was CE-certified in 2017 for commercial use in the European Union (EU). Eyemate has eight pressure and temperature sensors, designed for implantation in the ciliary sulcus at the time of cataract surgery [7].

Each pressure sensor has two parallel plates, the base plate is rigid while the plate that indents with changes in IOP is flexible. The distance between these two plates varies with fluctuations in IOP, generating an analog signal, which is then converted to a digital signal, that is transmitted to a small handheld mesograph by radiofrequency. For the reader to activate the electromagnetic coupling sequence and the units to correspond with each other, the reader and the intraocular transponder unit must be within 5 cm of each other. The device can obtain up to 10 IOP measurements per second. The Eyemate (with a GSM module) data can be shared with the physician using an internet database.

EYEMATE-SC when implanted in patients with primary open-angle glaucoma (POAG) undergoing simultaneous nonpenetrating glaucoma surgery (NPGS) was found to be safe and well tolerated through 12 months [8].

Literature reassures that the Smart IOP sensors hold promise for redefining glaucoma treatment strategies.

Digital photography:

Remote or rural areas have limited access to good ophthalmic care with the state-of-the-art diagnostic equipment, especially for detecting preperimetric or early glaucomatous damage [9]. Smartphone-based teleglaucoma screening can help in early detection and treatment.

Affordable adapters that convert a smartphone camera into a miniature anterior segment and fundus camera have flooded the markets globally.

Some of the adapters used in community studies include the Peek (Peek Vision; https://www.peekvision.org) from England, the D-Eye system (Si 14; https://www.d-eyecare.com) from Italy, and the IExaminer (Welch Allyn), EyeGo (Stanford University and DigiSight Technologies), and Ocular CellScope (University of California, Berkeley) from the United States.

These smart devices are being used to capture "direct" images or video of the posterior pole (in an undilated state, without the condensing +20 D lens) not only by the ophthalmologists and optometrists but also by the neurologists and paediatricians. These images can be shared for expert assessment (HIPPA compliant) and saved to a patient file for future reference [10, 11].

Results from Smartphone ophthalmoscopy has shown good agreement with slit lamp examination for the estimation of optic nerve head cupping or glaucoma detection [12].

B. **Perimetry:**

Tablet Perimetry: Mobile applications that allow visual field (VF) charting have opened up options for a small clinical setup or even home-based perimetry where standard automated perimetry (SAP). Several tools are available for VF charting on tablets, laptops, and desktop computers [13].

Melbourne Rapid Fields (MRF): MRF is an iPad tablet application (iPad 3 or later) that allows in-office or remote VF testing [14].

Recently, an Online website version of MRF has been made available that has a web-cam technology to monitor viewing distance as well as gaze stability. Online version can be accessed at the webpage, www.visioninhome.com.

MRF Glaucoma detects VF abnormalities both centrally as well as peripherally (up to 30° from central fixation point). At the end of each test, longitudinal comparison of test results is performed. Stored test results can be accessed through an online portal, exported as comma separated values (.CVS) format and imported into Excel for detailed point-to-point analysis. User experience using MRF has been positive [15].

Prea SM et al. have shown that MRF correlated strongly with SAP using Humphrey visual field analyser (HFA), over a 6-month period across four visits, with good test-retest reliability [16].

It is important to remember that although the average mean deviation (MD) values from MRF or a Smart Visual Function Analyzer (SVFA) such as IMOvifa™ provide similar results to the HFA, point-by-point comparisons show notable deviations [17]. These differences could partly be due to the different normative databases as well as the difference in MD calculation. The tablet design itself may also account for variations in the local sensitivities.

Tablet perimetry has garnered interest during COVID and in the post COVID era as it can be done at home or in the waiting room, thus saving time [18].

C. **Contrast Sensitivity Testing:**

The Spaeth Richman Contrast Sensitivity Test (SPARCS): SPARCS helps assess both central as well as peripheral contrast sensitivity (CS) using the Weber contrast. The test requires internet access on a standard computer with monitor set to 1024 × 768 resolution, 256 grey levels and a size of at least 22 cm width and 26.5 cm height. The test is available at *https://www.sparcscontrastcenter.com*. The website provides instructions on how to take the test. Each patient gets a unique identification number. At a testing distance of 50 cms, the test occupies 30° of vision horizontally and 23.5° of vision vertically. The central test area subtends 3.5° vertically and 5° horizontally. Patient has to fixate on the central area of the testing screen and identify the areas, which appears different. When patient is ready, they click on the central area. In one of the five test areas, vertical square wave gratings with a spatial frequency of 0.4 cycles per degree randomly appear for 0.3 s. Temporarily, patients break fixation to select the area with the grating. Patient fixates again on the central area and clicks on the screen to activate the programme to show the next area with grating. Correct and incorrect responses are recorded until the software determines the contrast threshold in each area. The test takes 5–10 min per eye [19].

The contrast threshold is determined using a staircase strategy with reversals. Initial correct responses advance four levels until the patient gives an incorrect response. After the incorrect response, a contrast level two levels easier than the previous one is presented. The algorithm advances or regresses one level at a time until two incorrect responses are made at a specific level, which establishes the contrast threshold. If a patient stops trying to guess the correct area and clicks the same location repeatedly, the test terminates. Patient is instructed to attempt to choose the location where the gratings appear. The range of contrast tested is from 100% to 0.45% (log contrast sensitivity 0.00–2.35) and decreases by approximately 0.15 log units between levels. The central area (CC) and four peripheral areas (SN, ST, IN, IT) each receive separate scores. A total SPARCS score is summated from each of the five areas (20 per area), resulting in a perfect score of 100.

Richman et al. studied the performance of SPARCS for glaucoma patients, and found that a total SPARCS score of <70 had a sensitivity of 79.7% and specificity of 92.8% in the identification of glaucoma in Caucasian population [19]. Thakur et al. have also found SPARCS to be a sensitive and reliable indicator of glaucomatous damage [20]. SPARCS has also been used to test CS in patients with refractive errors, cataract, age-related macular degeneration and idiopathic intracranial hypertension [21–23].

D. **Electrophysiology:**

nGoggle™: The nGoggle™ is a "virtual reality" (VR) goggle with embedded EEG sensors. It is a brain–computer interface platform (BCIP) for detecting and monitoring neurodegenerative diseases of eye and brain. It allows detection of steady-state visual evoked potentials (SSVEP) corresponding to pattern reversal visual stimuli [24].

A trial (NCT03760055) is ongoing to assess the ability of the nGoggle to detect VF loss in patients with glaucoma, as well as to differentiate different severity stages of glaucoma, its repeatability and reliability for patient self-testing and patient satisfaction compared to SAP, optical coherence tomography (OCT) metrics and Diopsys NOVA (Diopsys, Inc.).

Pattern Electroretinogram (PERG):

PERG measures the activity of retinal ganglion cells (RGCs) and possibly detects the early functional abnormalities in glaucoma. Available commercial devices include Diopsys' Nova and Argos Vision Testing Systems and Konan Medical's EvokeDx [25].

Steady-state PERG amplitude has been shown to progressively decrease over time in a subset of glaucoma suspects, with relatively steeper slope in treated compared to untreated glaucoma suspects [26]. EvokeDx device has been found to be useful to help assess central vision and evaluate damage to magnocellular (MC) pathway, however it is noncontributory in mapping specific structural changes or peripheral defects [27].

3 Newer Drugs

A. **Rho Kinase Inhibitors:** The two Rho kinase isoforms (ROCK 1 and ROCK 2) are the effectors for the Rho A, B, and C. These G proteins get activated after binding to guanosine triphosphate (GTP). Rho kinase inhibitors have a dual mechanism of action, increase in aqueous outflow, along with decrease in aqueous outflow resistance by increasing the pores formed by the endothelial cells in the Schlemm's canal (SC). They also increase the outflow by relaxing smooth muscle fibres of the trabecular meshwork (TM). In addition, Netarsudil has norepinephrine transporter (NET) inhibitor activity further lowers aqueous humour production as well as the episcleral venous pressure. Rho kinase may also be neuroprotective, possibly via increased optic nerve head perfusion, and may decrease postsurgical scarring. The latter action is because ROCK inhibitors inhibit fibroblasts activation via TGF-beta [2, 28].

   The two commonly used ROCK inhibitors are Ripasudil and Netarsudil. Ripasudil hydrochloride hydrate (Glanatec®) 0.4% which requires twice a day dosing and Netarsudil (Rhopressa®) 0.02% which is used once at bedtime [2]. They are both known to effective in lowering IOP in POAG and OHTN alike, with the most common side effects being conjunctival hyperaemia (75%), blepharitis (20%), and cornea verticillata (15%), with the latter being unique to Netarsudil.

   The fixed drug combination (FDC) of netarsudil 0.02% and latanoprost 0.005% (ROCKLATAN®) once daily has been found to resulted in greater mean IOP reduction as compared to monotherapy with either drug [29].

   The newest ROCK inhibitor in pipeline, Fasudil, has shown good IOP lowering even in end-stage glaucoma [30]. Use of depot formulation of Fasudil loaded polylactide-*co*-glycolide (PLGA) microspheres have been proposed in the form of intravitreal injection for glaucoma patients with coexistent retinal disease [31].

   Rho kinase inhibitors hold great promise as an adjunctive therapy, since their mechanism of action is different from the existing AGMs. Although adverse events, especially conjunctival hyperaemia and subconjunctival haemorrhages, may impact compliance in the long term, this class of AGM is a significant addition to the glaucoma practitioners armamentarium.

B. **Latanoprostene Bunod:** Latanoprostene bunod 0.024% (Vyzulta®) is a prodrug, which has the unique property of donating nitric oxide (NO). The drug metabolizes into latanoprost acid, and butanediol mononitrate; and the latter is further metabolized to 1,4-butanediol and NO.

   Latanoprost acid increases uveoscleral outflow via the Prostaglandin F receptor. Like all other prostaglandin agonists, it modulates the remodelling of the extracellular matrix of the ciliary muscle via matrix metalloproteinases. Nitric oxide, the second active metabolite of the prodrug, causes vasodilation and smooth muscle cell relaxation in the TM and SC by decreasing cell contractility and volume, thus increasing outflow facility [32]. LBN has shown to increase both, optic nerve head capillary blood volume and oxygen saturation more than latanoprost [33].

   The once daily dosing of LBN has been found to be more effective than both latanoprost and timolol. The most common side effects include conjunctival hyperemia (17%), eyelash growth (16%), irritation and pain (10%). LBN has been found to be as effective as netarsudil as an adjuvant therapy [34].

C. **Novel Methods of Drug Delivery**

Nanotechnology: Nanotechnology-based treatments may improve patient quality of life, and consequently adherence, because of targeted drug delivery, better bioavailability, sustained release of the AGM or anti-metabolite (in case of glaucoma surgeries), and better therapeutic efficiency [35].

Additionally, nanomedicine formulations may have decreased side effects due to less frequent dosing [36]. These include liposomes, nanogels, nanoparticles, micelles, nanosuspensions, dendritic polymers, microneedles, etc., all of which have a particle size ranging from 1 to 100 nm, have shown to have significantly better therapeutic safety and efficacy than conventional ophthalmic formulations in animal studies. Even though this is yet to be a part of clinical practice, nanomedicine formulations of several AGMs that have been tried include supraciliary injection of brimonidine-laden microspheres, subconjunctival injection of dorzolamide nanoparticles and intravitreal injection of brimonidine, travoprost, and bimatoprost-laden nanosponges [2, 37, 38].

Implants:

Antiglaucoma drugs dispensed as injectable systems and undertrial punctal plug delivery systems are enlisted in Table 1.

(a) ***Bimatoprost implant:*** The bimatoprost implant (Durysta™) is a sustained release, biodegradable implant uses the NOVADUR drug delivery system. A 28-gauge, prefilled applicator releases this implant intracamerally. The biodegradable polymers of the implant disintegrate within the anterior chamber into carbon dioxide and water. The main adverse event noted was conjunctival hyperemia in almost one in three patients, and a more than

Table 1 Antiglaucoma drugs dispensed as Injectable systems and Undertrial Punctal plug delivery systems

Drug delivery system	Drug	Material	Placement of location	Current stage of development
ENV515/PGA or Travoprost XR	Travoprost	–	Anterior chamber angle	Phase 2 clinical trial
Bimatoprost SR	Bimatoprost	–	Subconjunctival space	Phase 3 clinical trial
Graybug	Various	–	Ocular surface	Preclinical
OTX-TP	Travoprost	Polyethylene glycol-based hydrogel with loaded PLA	Puncta	Phase 2 clinical trial
Evolute	Latanoprost	–	Puncta	Phase 2 clinical trial
Latanoprost punctal plug delivery system (L-PPDS)	Latanoprost	–	Puncta	Phase 2 clinical trial

20% reduction in endothelial cell density in 10% and 21% of the 10 and 15 mcg groups. About 4% and 10% of eyes in each of the two groups, respectively, needed implant removal because of the corneal oedema, in order to prevent further endothelial loss. Better formulations are currently under review [39, 40].

(b) ***BIM ring:*** The bimatoprost ocular ring (Bimatoprost HELIOS™ insert, Abbvie) is a silicone—polypropylene ring impregnated with bimatoprost (24–29 mm in diameter) which is inserted in the fornices. It provides sustained IOP control over 6 months, eluting 6–35 microns of the drug per day. The device does not have FDA approved yet [41].

(c) ***Travoprost punctum plugs:*** Recently, Polyethylene glycol resorbable hydrogel punctal plugs impregnated with travoprost, OTX-TP (Ocular Therapeutix, Inc.) have been developed. The retention rates of these plugs were 90% at 2 months, but less than 50% at 3 months. The other major adverse event reported was foreign body sensation in almost 40% patients, with the tolerability increasing over time [42].

Precise targeted delivery will minimize drug wastage by preventing drug loss due to systemic absorption and first-pass metabolism. High prevalence of ocular surface disease in patients instilling AGMs with added preservatives may be overcome with the newer devices [43].

4 Visual Rehabilitation

(a) **Virtual reality based low vision aids:** For patients with advanced glaucoma using low vision aids, augmented reality magnification can be done with devices such as Microsoft HoloVision Hololens and a camera worn on the finger [44].

Electronic head-mounted low vision aid (e-LVA) SightPlus (GiveVision, UK, givevision.net) improves visual function in people with low vision [45].

(b) **Smartphone applications for people with low vision:** Several smartphone apps are available that can make day-to-day tasks easier for people with visual impairment to improve their quality of life [46].
   - **NavCog:** This iPhone based app is helpful for indoor navigation, inside complex building spaces such as an airport or hospital. (*https://www.cs.cmu.edu/~NavCog/navcog.html*)
   - **Seeing AI:** This app gives a narration of the surrounding world around the patient through their phone's camera. It can help to identify and describes people, objects (e.g., currency) and documents (reads them aloud). Additionally, it can describe features such as colour, light, and handwriting.
   - In future, patients can get customized digital devices and apps to address their low vision.
   - We are hopeful that the emerging technologies will not only help mitigate the disease but also improve the quality of life of those with advanced or end stage glaucoma.

References[1]

1. Twa MD. Advances in glaucoma management. Optom Vis Sci. 2020;97(2):53.
2. Mohan N, Chakrabarti A, Nazm N, Mehta R, Edward DP. Newer advances in medical management of glaucoma. Indian J Ophthalmol. 2022;70(6):1920–30.
3. Cvenkel B, Velkovska MA, Jordanova VD. Self-measurement with Icare HOME tonometer, patients' feasibility and acceptability. Eur J Ophthalmol. 2020;30(2):258–63.
4. Takagi D, Sawada A, Yamamoto T. Evaluation of a new rebound self-tonometer, Icare HOME. J Glaucoma. 2017;l26(7):613–8.
5. Barbour-Hastie CC, Tatham AJ. Teaching home tonometry using a remote video link. Eye (Lond). 2023;37(3):501–5.
6. Yang C, Huang X, Li X, Yang C, Zhang T, Wu Q, Liu D, Lin H, Chen W, Hu N, Xie X. Wearable and implantable intraocular pressure biosensors: recent progress and future prospects. Adv Sci (Weinheim). 2021;8(6):2002971.
7. Enders P, Cursiefen C. Device profile of the EYEMATE-IO™ system for intraocular pressure monitoring: overview of its safety and efficacy. Expert Rev Med Devices. 2020;17(6):491–7.
8. Szurman P, Gillmann K, Seuthe AM, Dick HB, Hoffmann EM, Mermoud A, Mackert MJ, Weinreb RN, Rao HL, Mansouri K, EYEMATE-SC Study Group. EYEMATE-SC trial: twelve-month safety, performance, and accuracy of a suprachoroidal sensor for telemetric measurement of intraocular pressure. Ophthalmology. 2023;130(3):304–12.
9. Morjaria P, Bergson S, Bastawrous A, Watts E, Pant S, Gudwin E, Zinn M, Chan VF. Delivering refractive care to populations with near and distance vision impairment: 2 novel social enterprise models. Asia Pac J Ophthalmol. 2022;11(1):59–65.
10. Andersen T, Jeremiah M, Thamane K, Littman-Quinn R, Dikai Z, Kovarik C, Ndlovu K. Implementing a school vision screening program in Botswana using smartphone technology. Telemed J E Health. 2020;26(2):255–8.
11. Shukla K, Sapkota YD, Das AV, Morjaria P. Communication technology for eye care. Community Eye Health. 2022;35(114):1–2.
12. Russo A, Mapham W, Turano R, Costagliola C, Morescalchi F, Scaroni N, Semeraro F. Comparison of smartphone ophthalmoscopy with slit-lamp biomicroscopy for grading vertical cup-to-disc ratio. J Glaucoma. 2016;25(9):e777–81.
13. Prager AJ, Kang JM, Tanna AP. Advances in perimetry for glaucoma. Curr Opin Ophthalmol. 2021;32(2):92–7.
14. Harris PA, Johnson CA, Chen Y, Fann H, Gafford G, Kim YJ, Mezgebu ED. Evaluation of the Melbourne rapid fields test procedure. Optom Vis Sci. 2022;99(4):372–82.
15. Kumar H, Thulasidas M. Comparison of perimetric outcomes from Melbourne rapid fields tablet perimeter software and Humphrey field analyzer in glaucoma patients. J Ophthalmol. 2020;2020:8384509.
16. Prea SM, Kong YXG, Mehta A, He M, Crowston JG, Gupta V, Martin KR, Vingrys AJ. Six-month longitudinal comparison of a portable tablet perimeter with the Humphrey field analyzer. Am J Ophthalmol. 2018;190:9–16.
17. Kang J, De Arrigunaga S, Freeman SE, Zhao Y, Lin M, Liebman DL, Roldan AM, Kim JA, Chang DS, Friedman DS, Elze T. Comparison of perimetric outcomes from a tablet perimeter, smart visual function analyzer, and Humphrey field analyzer. Ophthalmol Glaucoma. 2023;6:S2589–4196(23)00059–5.
18. Ichhpujani P, Dhillon H. Spotlight on iPad visual field tests efficacy. Clin Ophthalmol. 2022;16:2179–85.

[1] **Note: Some text is taken from the author's previously published chapter in a book which is part of the same series.** *Ichhpujani, P.* (2020). Recent advances in glaucoma diagnostics. In: Ichhpujani, P. (*eds*) Current advances in ophthalmic technology. Current Practices in Ophthalmology. Springer, Singapore. https://doi.org/10.1007/978-981-13-9795-0_4

19. Richman J, Zangalli C, Lu L, Wizov SS, Spaeth E, Spaeth GL. The Spaeth/Richman contrast sensitivity test (SPARCS): design, reproducibility and ability to identify patients with glaucoma. Br J Ophthalmol. 2015;99(1):16–20.
20. Thakur S, Ichhpujani P, Kumar S, et al. Assessment of contrast sensitivity by Spaeth Richman contrast sensitivity test and Pelli Robson Chart Test in patients with varying severity of glaucoma. Eye (Lond). 2018;32:1392–400.
21. Faria BM, Duman F, Zheng CX, Waisbourd M, Gupta L, Ali M, Zangalli C, Lu L, Wizov SS, Spaeth E, Richman J, Spaeth GL. Evaluating contrast sensitivity in age-related macular degeneration using a novel computer-based test, the Spaeth/Richman contrast sensitivity test. Retina. 2015;35(7):1465–73.
22. Gupta L, Cvintal V, Delvadia R, Sun Y, Erdem E, Zangalli C, Lu L, Wizov SS, Richman J, Spaeth E, Spaeth GL. SPARCS and Pelli-Robson contrast sensitivity testing in normal controls and patients with cataract. Eye (Lond). 2017;31(5):753–61.
23. Ichhpujani P, Thakur S, Spaeth GL. Contrast sensitivity and glaucoma. J Glaucoma. 2020;29(1):71–5.
24. Nakanishi M, Wang YT, Jung TP, Zao JK, Chien YY, Diniz-Filho A, Daga FB, Lin YP, Wang Y, Medeiros FA. Detecting glaucoma with a portable brain-computer interface for objective assessment of visual function loss. JAMA Ophthalmol. 2017;135(6):550–7.
25. Al-Nosairy KO, Hoffmann MB, Bach M. Non-invasive electrophysiology in glaucoma, structure and function-a review. Eye (Lond). 2021;35(9):2374–85.
26. Gordon PS, Kostic M, Monsalve PF, Triolo G, Golubev L, Luna G, Ventura LM, Feuer WJ, Porciatti V. Long-term PERG monitoring of untreated and treated glaucoma suspects. Doc Ophthalmol. 2020;141(2):149–56.
27. https://www.aao.org/eyenet/article/does-perg-have-a-role-in-the-glaucoma-clinic. Accessed 11 Sept 2023.
28. Freiberg JC, von Spreckelsen A, Kolko M, Azuara-Blanco A, Virgili G. Rho kinase inhibitor for primary open-angle glaucoma and ocular hypertension. Cochrane Database Syst Rev. 2022;6(6):CD013817.
29. Asrani S, Bacharach J, Holland E, McKee H, Sheng H, Lewis RA, Kopczynski CC, Heah T. Fixed-dose combination of netarsudil and latanoprost in ocular hypertension and open-angle glaucoma: pooled efficacy/safety analysis of phase 3 MERCURY-1 and -2. Adv Ther. 2020;37(4):1620–31.
30. Pakravan M, Beni AN, Ghahari E, Varshochian R, Yazdani S, Esfandiari H, Ahmadieh H. The ocular hypotensive efficacy of topical fasudil, a rho-associated protein kinase inhibitor, in patients with end-stage glaucoma. Am J Ther. 2017;24(6):e676–80.
31. Mietzner R, Kade C, Froemel F, Pauly D, Stamer WD, Ohlmann A, Wegener J, Fuchshofer R, Breunig M. Fasudil loaded PLGA microspheres as potential intravitreal depot formulation for glaucoma therapy. Pharmaceutics. 2020;12(8):706.
32. Drugs and Lactation Database (LactMed®) [Internet]. Bethesda (MD): National Institute of Child Health and Human Development; 2006. Latanoprostene Bunod. 2022. PMID: 30000019.
33. Samaha D, Diaconu V, Bouchard JF, Desalliers C, Dupont A. Effect of latanoprostene bunod on optic nerve head blood flow. Optom Vis Sci. 2022;99(2):172–6.
34. Lo TC, Chen YY, Hung MC, Chou P. Latanoprostene bunod 0.024% in the treatment of open-angle glaucoma and ocular hypertension: a meta-analysis. J Clin Med. 2022;11(15):4325.
35. Occhiutto ML, Maranhão RC, Costa VP, Konstas AG. Nanotechnology for medical and surgical glaucoma therapy-a review. Adv Ther. 2020;37(1):155–99.
36. El Hoffy NM, Abdel Azim EA, Hathout RM, Fouly MA, Elkheshen SA. Glaucoma: management and future perspectives for nanotechnology-based treatment modalities. Eur J Pharm Sci. 2021;158:105648.
37. Cardigos J, Ferreira Q, Crisóstomo S, Moura-Coelho N, Cunha JP, Pinto LA, Ferreira JT. Nanotechnology-ocular devices for glaucoma treatment: a literature review. Curr Eye Res. 2019;44(2):111–7.
38. Wu Y, Tao Q, Xie J, Lu L, Xie X, Zhang Y, Jin Y. Advances in nanogels for topical drug delivery in ocular diseases. Gels. 2023;9(4):292.

39. 18 month prospective efficacy and safety study of bimatoprost intracameral implant (DURYSTA). ClinicalTrials.gov. Identifier: NCT04647214. https://clinicaltrials.gov/ct2/show/NCT04647214. Accessed 1 May 2023
40. Craven ER, Walters T, Christie WC, Day DG, Lewis RA, Goodkin ML, et al. 24 month phase I/ II clinical trial of bimatoprost sustained release implant (Bimatoprost SR) in glaucoma patients. Drugs. 2020;80:167–79.
41. Brandt JD, DuBiner HB, Benza R, Sall KN, Walker GA, Semba CP, Collaborators. Long-term safety and efficacy of a sustained-release bimatoprost ocular ring. Ophthalmology. 2017;124(10):1565–6.
42. Perera SA, Ting DS, Nongpiur ME, Chew PT, Aquino MC, Sng CC, Ho SW, Aung T. Feasibility study of sustained-release travoprost punctum plug for intraocular pressure reduction in an Asian population. Clin Ophthalmol. 2016;10:757–64.
43. Singh RB, Ichhpujani P, Thakur S, Jindal S. Promising therapeutic drug delivery systems for glaucoma: a comprehensive review. Ther Adv Ophthalmol. 2020;12:2515841420905740.
44. Kinateder M, Gualtieri J, Dunn MJ, Jarosz W, Yang XD, Cooper EA. Using an augmented reality device as a distance-based vision aid-promise and limitations. Optom Vis Sci. 2018;95(9):727–37.
45. Crossland MD, Starke SD, Imielski P, Wolffsohn JS, Webster AR. Benefit of an electronic head-mounted low vision aid. Ophthalmic Physiol Opt. 2019;39(6):422–31.
46. https://www.aao.org/eye-health/tips-prevention/low-vision-impairment-apps-tech-assistive-devices. Accessed 11 Sept 2023.

Advances in the Management of Oculomotor Dysfunction in Adults and Children with Concussion

Tiong Peng Yap and Cathy Stern

1 Vision and Concussion

Mild traumatic brain injury (TBI) arising from a bump, blow, shake or jolt to the head or body is often referred to as a concussion [1]. Approximately, 70–80% of all TBIs are classified as mild in the absence of lesions from brain imaging and/or loss of consciousness. This may arise from road traffic accidents, falls, sports injuries, assaults, recreational activities, or children's playground accidents. For example, sudden rapid changes in movement during whiplash can cause the brain to bounce, stretch or twist within the skull. This neurological event may result in focal and/or diffuse damage to neuronal dendrites, axons, and astrocytes, disrupting cellular membranes and releasing neurotransmitters. This invariably affects the intracellular and extracellular ionic equilibrium which consequently cause neuroinflammation and cell loss [2].

Concussion patients may suffer from a wide range of issues, given the pervasiveness of the injury. This includes sensory, motor, perceptual, cognitive, attentional, behavioral, somatic, academic, linguistic, and social well-being issues. Oculomotor, vestibular, and visual processing disorders are frequently experienced. Thus, it is necessary to investigate each of these functions carefully so that the appropriate treatment, therapy, and rehabilitation can be rendered to the patient.

The terms 'oculomotor' and 'ocular motor' tend to be used interchangeably in the literature despite their contextual differences in terms of nerve innervations and eye movements respectively. Although the latter is more accurate, it is more common to use the term 'oculomotor' to describe eye movement function or disorders.

T. P. Yap (✉)
IGARD Vision Therapy Center, Singapore, Singapore
e-mail: tiongyap@igard.com.sg

C. Stern
Pappas Rehabilitation Hospital for Children, Canton, MA, USA

D. Shu et al. (eds.), *Current Advances in Optometry*, Current Practices in Ophthalmology, https://doi.org/10.1007/978-981-97-8140-9_5

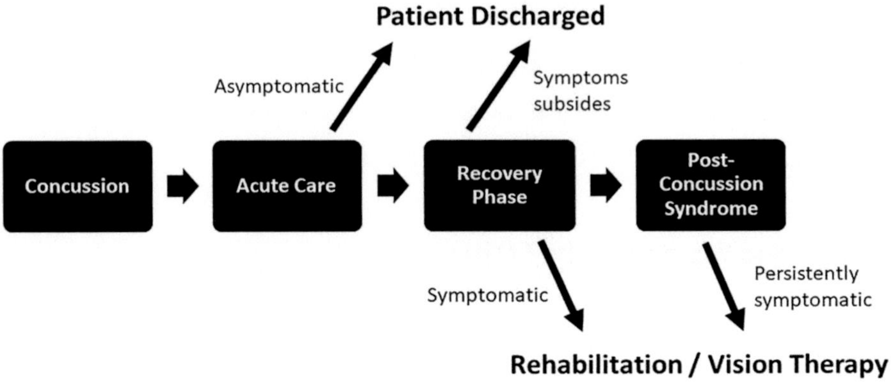

Fig. 1 Clinical management of concussion patients

1.1 Acute Care of the Concussion Patient

Acute care of the concussion patient typically involves management of symptoms (Fig. 1) and evaluating the likelihood of an intracranial injury based on the symptoms reported by the patient and/or brain imaging. To satisfy the diagnostic criteria of concussion, the Glasgow coma score should be 13–15, or any loss of consciousness should be less than 30 min and/or amnesia should be less than 24 h.

Given the high risks during sports, any symptoms, physical signs, and/or alterations of cognitive functioning may indicate a concussion in athletes [3]. In pediatric patients, age-appropriate concussion symptom scales are available [1] and additional signs should be taken into consideration, such as loss of appetite, refusal to engage in routine activities, and/or increased dependence on parents.

1.2 Recovery of the Concussion Patient

Relative Rest is important for brain injury recovery. Rest during the recovery phase allows inflammation to reduce and the brain to recover. If the condition is not worsening, concussion patients are often discharged from hospitals and encouraged to rest at home with limitations of activities involving mental concentration (e.g., video games and reading) and physical exertion (e.g. sports) to allow the symptoms to subside. After the first few days, one should gradually increase physical activity to a level that does not provoke symptoms. The duration for recovery depends on age [4], gender [5], severity [6], and presence of comorbid conditions, such as migraines, mood, learning, and attention-deficit disorders [1].

While full recovery is generally expected within weeks or up to 3 months, activities within the next 2–3 days should be light and kept to a level that does not provoke symptoms especially when returning-to-work (or school). To avoid the risk of a repeat concussion, return-to-sports (or play) should be conducted in a safe manner and guided using a graduated return-to-sport strategy [7] along with baseline measurements of neurocognitive function. However, patients with prolonged or persistent symptoms lasting weeks, months, or years [8] may require intervention as they are likely to have post-concussion syndrome.

1.3 Post-concussion Syndrome and Vision

Post-concussion syndrome refers to concussive symptoms that have lasted longer than expected. These may include headaches, blurred vision, double vision (diplopia), photosensitivity, nauseousness, dizziness, fogginess, and/or disequilibrium in busy environments.

Patients with oculomotor and/or vestibular dysfunction tend to be overwhelmed and cannot navigate in complex visual environments. They may present with visual motion sensitivity, visual-attentional deficits or visual field deficits. Some patients may present with gait or neurocognitive impairment. They may feel more emotional than usual or find it difficult to concentrate [7] and they may have heightened sensitivity to light or noise.

Post-concussion oculomotor dysfunction carries a four-times risk of developing chronic post-concussion syndrome [9]. Those who are symptomatic for 30 days or more tend to have significant challenges in vision and concentration [10]. Particularly in children and adolescents, nearly 14% remain symptomatic after 3 months [6] which adversely impacts reading, daily work, school or play activities.

Long-term repetitive concussion may contribute to mood or personality changes (e.g., depression), attention-deficit, hyperactivity, and anxiety disorders [11] and can potentially result in chronic traumatic encephalopathy. Therefore, it is essential to investigate oculomotor and vestibular functions carefully in order to facilitate the appropriate referral for vision therapy or Neuro Optometric Rehabilitation Therapy.

2 Oculomotor Dysfunction in Concussion

Oculomotor dysfunction affects more than 60% of concussed children and adolescents [12] and more than 90% of concussed adults [13]. Deficits in saccades, smooth pursuit, vergence, and accommodation are frequently observed [14]. In the absence of symptoms or in situations where patients are unable to recall the concussion, oculomotor function may be used as an objective biomarker in early detection [15] and for monitoring recovery [14].

The propensity for the visual system to be affected may be related to the large extent of the human brain involved in visual processing. As discussed previously, 'ocular motor function' describes the overall quality of eye movement but 'oculomotor dysfunction' is the term more commonly used in the literature to describe eye movement disorders. Thus, oculomotor function can be defined as the ability of the visual system to accurately fixate and track a moving target or when the person is moving; and to keep the target clearly in focus at all times. This entire process relies

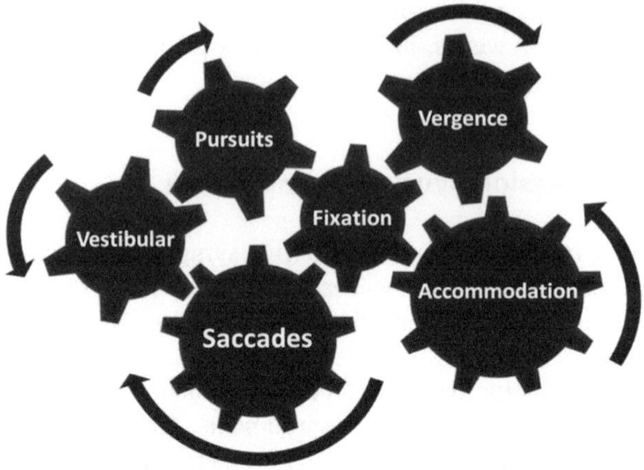

Fig. 2 Schematic representation of the neurological elements that mediates oculomotor function

on the visual system's capacity to align the eyes accurately in relation to the vestibular and proprioceptive systems.

Screening tools, such as the Vestibular Ocular Motor Screening (VOMS), King-Devick test or computerized eye tracker protocols can be used for initial diagnosis of oculomotor dysfunction but should by followed by a complete neuro optometric evaluation. The evaluation provides more detailed information about the oculomotor dysfunction, including the fixation, accommodation, vergence, saccadic eye movements, smooth pursuit eye movements and vestibular-oculomotor function (Fig. 2). Each of these visual functions may be considered as a neurological element that mediates oculomotor function, where each of them tend to interact with another. For example, vergence and the accommodative systems are tightly coupled in the process in maintaining accurate fixation, while pursuit eye movements entails steady and accurate fixation in relation to the vestibular system in order to hold the gaze. Each of these neurological elements needs to be assessed carefully during the neuro optometric evaluation, so any deficits can be diagnosed and properly managed in a treatment plan.

2.1 Fixational Disorders

Fixational disorders can occur after a concussion, resulting in an inability to maintain a stable image on the fovea. Fixation or visual fixation refers to the ability to voluntarily maintain a steady and accurate eye position that is focused on a target in order to prevent attention from fading away.

As the foveal field covers only 2° of the visual fields of each eye, precise fixational eye movements are needed to prevent the visual images from "slipping" away from the fovea. Small slow drifts (amplitudes ranging 1.5–4 arc minutes), tremors (rapid oscillatory movements of approx. 200 Hz with amplitudes ranging 5–30 sec arc), and microsaccades (fast jerky involuntary eye movements with amplitudes ranging 10–12 arc minutes) are actively occurring to fine-tune and ensure an accurate fixation.

As interactions between fixational eye movements and directed visual attention are mediated in the median cingulate gyrus, frontal eye fields (FEFs) and supplementary eye fields (SEFs) [16], fixational disorders post-concussion can affect a person's visual attention in a similar way to the poor fixation linked to attention deficit hyperactivity disorder (ADHD) traits [17]. Previous experiments found that microsaccades can result in a gaze shift from a target to another location of interest if the fixation is poorly engaged [18], thus affecting visual attention, visual perception and cognition.

In addressing fixational disorders, two major neurological elements in the process of fixation must be considered—vergence and accommodation. These systems actively align and adjust the focus of each eye synchronously to maintain the fixation. Similarly, any microsaccades during each fixation are typically conjugate eye movements with equal velocity and amplitudes, so both accommodative and vergence systems are tightly coupled in the process of fixation. Therefore, both systems need to be carefully examined in concussion patients.

2.2 Accommodative Disorders

Accommodative disorders are estimated to affect nearly 50% of post-concussion adolescents and children [12, 19, 20]. Accommodation is the neurological process in maintaining a clear and sharp image on the retina while the distance of objects may vary anywhere from distance (infinity) to as close as approximately 6 cm from the eye depending on the patient's age and in the absence of presbyopia.

As part of a complex neural control system, the accommodative system responds to retinal image blur through a neural feedback mechanism and constantly fine tunes itself in order to maintain a clear image on the retina. The autonomic innervation of the ciliary smooth muscles during accommodation is principally mediated by a fast reflexive parasympathetic (~1 s) and a slow adaptive sympathetic nervous system (~10 s) which produces dynamic changes and sustained steady-state responses, respectively.

Patients with accommodative disorder may report headaches, blurred vision, eyestrain, nauseousness, dizziness, and visual fatigue. These symptoms are similar to the symptoms experienced by patients with convergence insufficiency. Both conditions can be present in patients demonstrating receded near point of convergence (NPC) [20]. In one study of 74 patients with receded NPC, 95% had oculomotor dysfunction, 41% accommodative disorders only, 28% convergence insufficiency and accommodative disorders, and 8% convergence insufficiency alone. Therefore, a thorough examination of the vergence and accommodative systems is essential for accurate diagnosis [20].

Accommodative disorders can be broadly classified into accommodative insufficiency and accommodative excess. There may also be cases of aniso- or unequal accommodation in both eyes after brain injury which results in differential deficits between the two eyes. Accommodative insufficiency refers to premature weakening or paralysis of the accommodative system that is not within age expected norms, whereas accommodative excess occurs when a disproportionately large magnitude of accommodation is used during a near task. In the latter situation, the actual accommodative response during a particular task tends to exceed the accommodative demand, leading to an overexertion of the ciliary muscles.

Accommodative excess may be seen with a vergence disorder where excessive accommodation may be exerted to reduce diplopia [21] or it may occur following a brain injury in the absence of vergence disorder resulting in an accommodative spasm [22]. Thus, the visual system may fail to relax accommodation readily and patients may complain of headaches after prolonged near work or experience blurred vision in the distance after prolonged periods of near work. In school-aged children, accommodative infacility may contribute to slowness in adjusting focus from distance to near or vice versa and may affect tasks such as copying from the board in school.

The extent of the accommodative insufficiency or excess can be assessed by measuring the amplitude of accommodation, determining if there is a lag or lead of accommodation and evaluating the speed taken in exerting and relaxing the ciliary muscles. Amplitude of accommodation should be measured by moving an accommodative target, e.g., a paragraph of N5 print, at 1–2 cm/s toward the eye with the endpoint being the first sustained blur. The neuro optometric evaluation entails quantitative and qualitative measures of accommodation with careful interpretation in relation to vergence and oculomotor function. For example, dynamic retinoscopy can be used to assess accommodative lead or lag with additional observation to determine if the accommodation is oscillating or is accurate and sustainable. Accommodative facility can be measured with alternation of ±2.00 lenses while viewing an accommodative target and noting the number of cycles per minute taken to regain clear vision.

To probe the accommodative response, positive and negative relative accommodation (PRA, NRA) can be measured to determine how the visual system would respond to changes in the accommodative demand while vergence remains unchanged.

2.3 Vergence Disorders

Vergence disorders refer to a wide range of sensorimotor and visual perceptual abnormalities in relation to differences in the position of the two eyes. Convergence insufficiency is the most commonly reported vergence abnormality, ranging 38–49% in children [20, 23] and 44–47% in adults [19, 24]. Other common vergence disorders include convergence excess, divergence insufficiency, divergence excess and decompensated horizontal or vertical phorias.

Vergence adjustments are dynamic and can be horizontal, vertical, or torsional. The proper coordination and alignment of the eyes enables the visual system to accurately locate targets at different distances. Slight difference in the position of the two retinae (or retinal disparity) must be readily reconciled by an adequate vergence response in order to achieve sensory fusion. While viewing objects that are nearer or further away, convergence or divergence of the two eyes works synchronously with accommodation at all distances under the influence of the proprioceptive system which gives the internal awareness of space. Failure to maintain vergence can result in unstable binocular vision, diplopia, asthenopia and visual discomfort.

Approximately half of those affected by a receded NPC post-concussion tend to recover without intervention in 4.5 weeks [25], but some patients experience persistent abnormalities lasting several months or longer [26]. In children with persistent post-concussive symptoms lasting longer than 28 days, a receded NPC was observed in 89% of them [20].

In sports-related concussion, receded NPC (>6 cm) appears to be a reliable biomarker for prolonged recovery (e.g. 50 days) [27]. Symptoms of convergence insufficiency tend to be similar to that reported in patients with accommodative disorder [20]. Since vergence disorders can influence accommodation, both conditions are often present in patients demonstrating a receded NPC. Hence, patients should ideally receive a neuro optometric evaluation 4–5 weeks post-concussion when other conditions will have abated.

Typically, the NPC breakpoints are measured as the distance from the point of diplopia to the nasion (bridge of the nose) and the recovery point is when single vision is re-established as the target is backed away. However, NPC measurements can be confounded by the patient's poor misinterpretation of blur versus diplopia. Receded NPC tends to be more apparent using a line target on the RAF rule (e.g. Grafton Optical, Berkhamsted, UK) compared to a pencil tip or fingertip [28], or when the target speed is increased [29]. NPC measurements alone may not be sufficient when evaluating vergence disorders but should be used as a screening test prior to a referral for neuro optometric evaluation.

Other diagnostic factors of convergence insufficiency include a larger exophoria at near than far and inadequate positive fusional vergence at near. Exophoria refers to the tendency for the eyes to deviate outwards and is a common observation after a concussion; whereas fusional vergence measurements determine if the patient has the capacity to sustain binocular single vision as the examiner increases negative and positive vergence demands while the patient maintains a constant level of accommodation. This is collectively also known as binocularity, which has to be assessed carefully by a clinician with the relevant training in optometry. While these heterophoria measurements will determine the relative deviation of the eyes when the two eyes are dissociated, such as during the cover test, an experienced clinician must also consider the interplay and influence of accommodation, refractive correction, spectacle lens design, head posture, vestibular input, and the patient's vestibular status.

Stereopsis can be measured using commercially available tests, such as the Frisby stereotest (Stereotest Ltd., Oxfordshire, UK). Typically, positive and negative fusional vergence (PFV and NFV) ranges are measured at a fixed distance of 40 cm using a prism bar (base-out and base-in, respectively) by increasing its magnitude until the blur and break (diplopia) points are found and reducing the prism until the recovery (single vision) point. In a full binocular vision work-up, vergence facility can be measured by alternating a 3Δ base-in/12Δ base-out prism while fixating on an accommodative target at 40 cm in order to determine the number of cycles per minute the patient can achieve while gaining single and clear vision during each alternation of the prisms.

2.4 Saccadic Disorders

Saccadic disorders are estimated to occur in 20–30% of concussion patients [12, 13] and its associated impairments tend to be more apparent under conditions of high cognitive load, such as reading or when watching fast moving objects. For example, patients may lose their place when reading, skip or re-read lines of print, face difficulty with eye contact, and academic learning may be affected [10]. Other symptoms of saccadic disorders may include asthenopia, headaches, and dizziness.

Saccadic eye movements (or saccades) involves rapid changes in fixation while shifting the gaze. In general, the process of reading tends to involve small amplitudes of saccades whereas large amplitudes would typically be used during visual scanning tasks. Following a concussion, these tasks tend to become more difficult due to poorer accuracy (hypo- or hypermetric), slower velocities, increased latencies, longer duration, and smaller peak accelerations in the saccadic eye movements. Vergence disorders often occur together with saccadic dysfunction because these two systems tend to interact during eye movements and may affect attention after concussion [30].

The normal function of saccades is to scan the visual environment (e.g., visual search or free viewing) in order to capture the image of interest as quickly as possible onto the fovea where photoreceptor density and visual resolution are the highest. Saccades can be voluntary or reflexive to visual, auditory, memory, and tactile stimuli. In response to changes in fixations, the eyes shift rapidly with a velocity of 400–800°/s from one object of fixation to another. This movement is brief (short duration of 10–100 ms), conjugate (i.e., parallel and same direction), and ballistic (i.e., unable to change the course of the eye movement without making a separate saccade).

Clinical examination typically evaluates the accuracy, latency, and velocity of the saccadic eye movements by asking the patient to alternately fixate between two targets 30–40° apart at a viewing distance of 40 cm. Latencies of 180–200 ms are normally observed at the beginning of a saccade, then it tends to be slightly hypometric (i.e., undershoot the target) by approximately 10% less than the amplitude of the intended target and is fine-tuned by a microsaccade. Reading-related eye movement can be examined using standardized rapid number naming tests, such as the Developmental Eye Movement (DEM) test (Bernell Corp., Mishawaka, Indiana, USA), or the King-Devick test (King-Devick Technologies Inc., Downers Grove, Illinois, USA). The latter is increasingly used in baseline testing and for sideline testing when subclinical concussions are suspected among athletes [31].

2.5 Smooth Pursuit Eye Movement Disorders

Smooth pursuit eye movement (SPEM) disorders are estimated to affect 43–60% of patients with concussion [14]. They tend to induce visual motion sensitivity, dizziness, and nausea when viewing objects in motion. This is largely because the eyes tend to lose track when unable to keep up with their speed, thus putting an additional load in the saccadic, vestibular, and optokinetic systems. This tends to elicit involuntary conjugate saccades that interrupt fixation knows as saccadic intrusions or a combination of eye and head movements in order to compensate or reduce that target error.

The fundamental purpose of SPEM is to assist with gaze holding where the two eyes produce conjugate movements (in the same direction) so the target remains accurately fixated on the fovea without head movement. While the neural process of gaze holding also involves the vestibular and optokinetic systems, SPEM maintains gaze accurately together with the fixational and vergence systems keeping it to a speed of 30–40°/s before shifting the gaze or moving the head. However, post-concussion SPEM can prove to be difficult for some patients as observed by their frequent fixations and saccades when tracking slow moving targets [32]. This affects their attention given that the prefrontal cortex is involved in both processes. For example, visual attention tends to be hindered when tracking multiple moving objects due to the increased tracking load and distraction [30].

Clinical evaluation of SPEM involves observing for smoothness, amplitude, velocity, and direction when the patient is following a 10–20°/s moving target, such as the tip of a pencil, at a distance of approximately 1 m. The patient should be instructed not to move his or her head, and the target should be moved in the vertical and horizontal planes. To track a moving object, a very quick "catch-up" saccade normally precedes the fixation and SPEM. Longer lags, smaller amplitudes, increased eye position errors, and variabilities in gaze positions may be observed post-concussion and SPEM may appear jerky due to saccadic intrusions and re-fixations. Alternatively, an optokinetic drum can be used to examine the patient's horizontal SPEM by following the alternating white and black vertical stripe patterns on the rotating drum. As the eyes moves toward the end of each excursion, a corrective saccade would be observed in the opposite direction—this normal phenomenon is known as optokinetic nystagmus and it relies on intact SPEM and saccadic systems in order to produce this normal rhythmic reflex response.

2.6 Vestibular-Ocular Disorders

Vestibular-ocular disorders are estimated to affect up to 71% of concussion patients [33]. This occurs when there is mismatched sensory-motor feedback from eye and head movements due to a disruption to the normal sensory integration of the visual and vestibular systems. This may produce a false sense of movement within the individual (internal vertigo), in the surroundings (oscillopsia or external vertigo), or a heightened sensitivity to head movement when shifting gaze. For example, a room may appear to be spinning, or there may be a sensation of falling, tilting or bouncing. These symptoms tend to exacerbate when there is an overreliance on the visual system or in visually complex environments, resulting in visual motion sensitivity and balance deficits in 40–68% of concussed patients [34]. Other symptoms include nausea, imbalance, dizziness, movement-related blurry vision, unsteadiness or anxiety in busy environments [34].

Vestibular brain injuries are generally classified as central (affecting the brain or central nervous system) or peripheral (pathology of inner ear vestibular structures and/or the vestibular portion of the eighth cranial nerve). Central vestibulopathy may result in disequilibrium and ataxia, which lead to difficulties in balance, coordination and walking. Peripheral vestibulopathy is most often due to benign paroxysmal positional vertigo (BPPV) which occurs when calcium carbonate crystals (otoconia) migrate from the utricle into the semi-circular canals. Some concussed patients develop temporary hearing loss due to labyrinthine concussion which occurs with or without BPPV.

While >90% of BPPV are successfully treated within weeks with canalith repositioning maneuver [35], patients with central vestibulopathy and/or vestibular-ocular disorders tend to have prolonged symptoms involving dizziness and visual instability which necessitates oculomotor and vestibular rehabilitation. This is because the vestibular system and the oculomotor functions are closely related. For example, the vestibulo-ocular reflex (VOR) is when the vergence and SPEM systems interact with the vestibular system during head movements in order to stabilize the eyes on a target relative to the external environment. Deficits in VOR can be accompanied with nystagmus. For example, patients with oscillopsia after moving the head often have positional nystagmus, whereas patients with oscillopsia unrelated to moving the head often acquire downbeat or pendular nystagmus which is characterized by slow upward followed by a fast downward drift of the eyes, or a fast sinusoidal oscillatory movement of the eyes respectively [36]. Therefore, it is important to examine the VOR in concussed patients with prolonged symptoms.

The VOR is mediated through the labyrinth of the inner ear (including the semicircular canals), vestibular nuclei and cerebellar flocculonodular lobe. There are two types of VORs: Firstly, angular VOR stabilizes vision during rotational acceleration using the semicircular canals. Secondly, translational VOR stabilizes vision during linear acceleration of the head and body using the otoliths (utricles and saccules). In the process of VOR, brief changes in head position would direct the eyes to move opposite the direction of head movement with equal amplitude in order to quickly correct the target error. This would allow the images to remain on the fovea and to process visual motion and motion parallax. In contrast, the VOR tends to be suppressed during large saccades as the head and eyes move in the same direction simultaneously. As the VOR may not respond to slow constant velocity motion and persistent rotation of the head, this situation then relies on the proprioceptive inputs from the neck.

In clinical practice, the head impulse test is used to evaluate VOR. While fixating on the examiner's nose or a distance target, the patient's head is quickly and unpredictably moved horizontally 20–30° by the examiner. The expected normal finding is a conjugate eye movement opposite direction of the head movement. The eyes should remain steadily fixated on the target during the neck rotation. Any refixation saccades would suggest that the VOR is abnormal. The patient's ability to suppress the VOR can be evaluated by asking the patient to fixate on the thumb of their outstretched arm while the chair is rotated, so any refixation saccades suggest an impaired ability to suppress the VOR. In addition, the patient should have their dynamic visual acuity examined after refraction and static visual acuity testing. This can be assessed by rotating the patient's head back and forth by 20–40° in the horizontal plane at approximately 2 Hz. As this head movement exceeds the ability of the pursuit system to compensate, a reduction of <2 lines in dynamic visual acuity is expected as compared to static visual acuity.

3 Treatment of Oculomotor Dysfunction in Concussion

It is essential for eye doctors to be able to initiate clinical management of visual symptoms given the prevalence of oculomotor dysfunction following a concussion. While estimates vary, a recent publication by the American Academy of Ophthalmology (AAO) referred to 69% of children and adolescents with a concussion having at least one associated vision disorder. The most common presenting vision disorders are convergence insufficiency, accommodative insufficiency, and saccadic dysfunction [37].

Treatment should be directed at full rehabilitation of the specific type of oculomotor dysfunction and the specific type of visual disorder affecting the patient. When a full recovery is not possible, compensatory or therapeutic interventions that reduces the symptoms should be included in the treatment plan.

The following are the most common interventions:

- Refractive correction
- Therapeutic lenses for symptom relief, or to assist focus flexibility or binocularity
- Prism lenses for spatial orientation, binocular compensation, balance, or postural control
- Spectral filters (color or tint) for light sensitivity or reading disability
- Selective occlusion for strabismus or diplopia
- Neuro Optometric Rehabilitation Therapy to remediate oculomotor dysfunction, inclusive of fixation, pursuits, saccades, accommodation, vergence, and binocularity.

While not being covered here, patients may also benefit from visual field expanding devices for visual field constriction or loss, optical devices for sight loss, non-optical aids for low vision or reading disability, and proper management or monitoring of eye disease.

The use of lenses, prisms, selective occlusion, and spectral filters or tints is integral to treating post-concussion syndrome. The goal of the treatment is to alleviate symptoms, achieve desired visual outcomes, meet the patient's needs, and improve the patient's quality of life.

Neuro Optometric Rehabilitation Therapy may be considered at the same time as the use of lenses, prisms, selective occlusion, and tints but may be needed alone or after a trial of these other more passive treatments. Here, the reasons or rationale of using each of these treatment modalities will be discussed.

3.1 Refractive Correction

Brain injury may change a patient's refractive status. A patient may need a change in spectacle prescription or a first prescription when they had no apparent prescriptive visual need prior to their injury. A patient wearing contact lenses may no longer be able to insert or remove the lenses and may not have a current eyeglasses prescription. They may have only worn spectacles for brief periods of time for many years and will therefore need a careful refraction that they can tolerate.

The prescription should consider both maximizing sight and patient comfort. If there is a significant difference in the spherical or cylindrical components between the two eyes, consider reducing the prescription in one eye to better balance the prescription. In clinical practice, if at least one meridian of the astigmatic prescription is equal between the two eyes, the patient can better tolerate wearing the prescription and there is little to no compromise of binocular eyesight or binocular vision status [38].

Trial frame testing should be considered with every patient. If the refraction is done in a phoropter, the desired prescription should be placed into a trial frame and the patient allowed to walk around with it on for a few minutes. Giving them the experience of near and far viewing along with body movement can be very helpful in knowing if the patient is likely to tolerate the new prescription in everyday activities.

3.2 Therapeutic Lenses

Therapeutic lenses can be prescribed for symptomatic relief, focus flexibility or to assist binocularity. Accommodative disorders are common after brain injury and a patient may benefit from a lens prescription for near-centered work, such as while reading or working at their computer. This is especially true for patients in their mid to late 30s who are approaching presbyopia. Brain injury places additional stress on a patient's system often leaving them stuck in a state of sympathetic fight or flight. Thus, these patients often benefit from low plus lenses of +0.25 to +0.50 OU during near-centered work. This not only reduces accommodative lag and accommodative demand, but can alter the perception of space to allow more "focalized" patients to better use their ambient vision and it helps to increase the VOR gain for those with vestibular issues.

3.3 Prism Lenses

Prism lenses can be prescribed to improve spatial orientation, binocular compensation, or postural control. The purpose is to bend the light entering the eye so that the image can be shifted in the direction of the prism apex, which may be more desirable for the neurological process. To reduce the convergence stress, small magnitude of bases in prisms (e.g., 1Δ before each eye) can be used for near-centered work to improve binocular stamina and stability.

Brain injured patients often compensate for visual information overload by constricting peripheral awareness (or ambient vision). Visual field testing often shows an overall constriction with no pathological pattern. Reduced peripheral awareness contributes to inaccurate eye movements, poor depth perception, convergence difficulty and poor eye-hand coordination. Thus, prescribing 1–2Δ bases down prism in each eye (yoked prism) can help to expand the patient's visual awareness which leads to greater binocular stability and increased patient safety as they go about their daily activities.

A third application of prisms can be for postural control. Given the non-uniform magnification of space across the visual field, prisms are able to produce spatial changes neurologically by countering the expansion or compression of space that is occurring in the ambient visual process. When a patient presents with limited head control, a head turn, or abnormal egocentric localization, vertical or horizontal yoked prism that is generally 3–4Δ per eye, may help the patient better center their visual world and therefore present with their head aligned and with improved head control.

3.4 Spectral Filters (Color or Tint) for Light Sensitivity or Reading Disability

Clinicians should be aware that a significant number of patients experience photosensitivity following brain injury, and some patients experience visual snow syndrome where tiny flickering dots can appear across the visual field. Spectral filters, or tinted lenses, can selectively eliminate visible wavelengths that are causing perceptual discomfort, visual snow, and reading disability [39].

While the exact hue and saturation level of these spectral filters can be precisely determined to ameliorate the symptoms of photosensitivity using an intuitive colorimeter (Cerium Visual Technologies Limited, Tenterden, Kent, UK), there is a series of recommended tints known as the Polytrauma Brain Injury Filter Kit available from Chadwick Optical (Pennsylvania, USA) (Table 1). Chadwick Optical surveyed clinicians from Veterans Affairs Polytrauma Centers as well as experienced doctors from the Neuro Optometric Rehabilitation Association (NORA, noravisionrehab.org) to develop the kit. While clinicians have had success with most of these tints, E-15, and FL 41 50% tend to be the ones most frequently chosen for indoor use and FL 27% (73% tint) for outdoor use.

Table 1 List of tinted ophthalmic lenses from the Polytrauma Brain Injury Filter Kit (Chadwick Optical: www.chadwickoptical.com)

Green/Blue	Plum
• Green/Blue 20%	• Light Plum (Noir 88)
• Blue/Green 20%	• Medium Plum (COI Plum)
Blue	• Dark Plum (Noir 81)
• E-15 Blue (Light Blue)	Rose
• E-30 Blue (Medium Blue)	• Light Rose (FL-41 75%)
• E-50 Blue (Dark Blue)	• Medium Rose (FL-41 50%)
• z1 Blue (Noir 26)	• Dark Rose (FL-41 27%)

3.5 Selective Occlusion

Patients do sometimes report diplopia that may be constant or intermittent. When lenses alone are not successful in relieving the diplopia, temporary occlusion may be needed. Contrary to traditional methods of occlusion, dark black "pirate" patches should not be used to cover one eye as they limit peripheral vision and therefore present a safety risk. Instead, occlusion that is opaque and only as broad as needed to reduce the diplopia is preferred. For example, even if a patient is highly sensitive to diplopia in all fields of gaze, consider placing opaque occlusion covering ¾ of one lens of a pair of spectacles, leaving the temporal portion of the lens clear, then adding nasal occlusion to the other spectacle lens if the patient still complains of diplopia when looking to the side of the lens that is already occluded.

Another approach commonly used in neuro optometric rehabilitation is to prescribe binasal occlusion, which can be useful in dampening the visual confusion that often arises in the area of greatest binocular overlap. In clinical practice, the authors' preference is to use Scotch® Removable Magic™ Tape or LP Bangerter occlusion foil which can be cut to size.

3.6 Neuro Optometric Rehabilitation Therapy

While many believe that neuro optometric rehabilitation is quite new, the concept of being able to rehabilitate or enhance oculomotor, accommodative and binocular vision skills has been in the literature since the nineteenth century. A French ophthalmologist, Louis Émile Javal, wrote his Manual of Strabismus in 1896 and is considered the father of orthoptics, a precursor to modern vision therapy and neuro optometric rehabilitation [40].

Neuro Optometric Rehabilitation Therapy is an individualized treatment program for patients with oculomotor deficits that either do not respond to other interventions or where the other interventions mentioned still leave them with residual deficits. There is evidence supporting vision therapy as an effective strategy for rehabilitation. For example, Ciuffreda, et al. found that treatment with eye tracking, accommodation and convergence exercises expedited recovery and completely alleviated symptoms in almost 90% of patients with mild TBI who have persistent oculomotor defects [41].

This therapy typically involves weekly in-office sessions with supportive home activities over an 8-month period until symptoms resolved [41]. This includes activities or techniques that are carefully planned and guided by eye doctors who are accredited or board certified in vision therapy and neuro optometric rehabilitation, so as to remediate the underlying neural deficits that limit oculomotor function. International accreditation bodies include the Neuro Optometric Rehabilitation Association (NORA), College of Optometrists in Vision Development (COVD)/Optometric Vision Development and Rehabilitation Association (OVDRA), Optometric Extension Program Foundation (OEPF), Australasian College of Behavioural Optometrists (ACBO), British Association of Behavioural Optometrists (BABO), and the Binocular Vision, Perception and Pediatric Optometry (BVPPO) Section of the American Academy of Optometry (AAO).

Typically, the therapy activities begin at a level where the patient can perform the activities without exacerbating their symptoms, and the level of the training activities is gradually increased according to the patient's response to the treatment. This helps in reducing the positional error of the eyes, reducing retinal slippage and improving gaze stability. The target distances and conditions of each activity are varied according to the treatment plan for the patient, with the goal being to normalize the sensorimotor deficits of binocular vision, improve visual perceptual skills, and integrate the oculomotor and vestibular systems. Techniques applicable to a neuro optometric rehabilitation program are available from resources, such as the Optometric Extension Program Foundation (OEPF) [42].

4 Summary

Oculomotor dysfunction affects more than 60% of concussed children and adolescents and more than 90% of concussed adults. Deficits in saccades, smooth pursuit, vergence, and accommodation are frequently observed. With proper refractive correction taking into account visual–vestibular interaction and the use of therapeutic lenses, prism lenses, spectral filters, selective occlusion, and/or a program of Neuro Optometric Rehabilitation Therapy, these patients will have their symptoms significantly or fully resolved and be able to return to their previous daily activities. Today, the eye and vision care community should recognize these post-concussion or mild brain injury visual issues and treat or refer these patients for what is considered the best medical care.

References

1. Lumba-Brown A, Yeates KO, Sarmiento K, et al. Diagnosis and management of mild traumatic brain injury in children: a systematic review. JAMA Pediatr. 2018;172:e182847.
2. Romeu-Mejia R, Giza CC, Goldman JT. Concussion pathophysiology and injury biomechanics. Curr Rev Musculoskelet Med. 2019;12:105–16.
3. McCrory P, Meeuwisse W, Johnston K, et al. Consensus statement on concussion in sport—the 3rd international conference on concussion in sport held in Zurich, November 2008. J Sci Med Sport. 2009;12:340–51.

4. Davis GA, Anderson V, Babl FE, et al. What is the difference in concussion management in children as compared with adults? A systematic review. Br J Sports Med. 2017;51:949–57.
5. Tanveer S, Zecavati N, Delasobera EB, Oyegbile TO. Gender differences in concussion and postinjury cognitive findings in an older and younger pediatric population. Pediatr Neurol. 2017;70:44–9.
6. Barlow KM, Crawford S, Stevenson A, Sandhu SS, Belanger F, Dewey D. Epidemiology of post-concussion syndrome in pediatric mild traumatic brain injury. Pediatrics. 2010;126:e374–81.
7. McCrory P, Meeuwisse W, Dvořák J, et al. Consensus statement on concussion in sport-the 5(th) international conference on concussion in sport held in Berlin, October 2016. Br J Sports Med. 2017;51:838–47.
8. Iverson GL. Outcome from mild traumatic brain injury. Curr Opin Psychiatry. 2005;18:301–17.
9. Master CL, Master SR, Wiebe DJ, et al. Vision and vestibular system dysfunction predicts prolonged concussion recovery in children. Clin J Sport Med. 2018;28:139–45.
10. Swanson MW, Weise KK, Dreer LE, et al. Academic difficulty and vision symptoms in children with concussion. Optom Vis Sci. 2017;94:60–7.
11. Ellis MJ, Cordingley D, Vis S, Reimer K, Leiter J, Russell K. Vestibulo-ocular dysfunction in pediatric sports-related concussion. J Neurosurg Pediatr. 2015;16:248–55.
12. Master CL, Scheiman M, Gallaway M, et al. Vision diagnoses are common after concussion in adolescents. Clin Pediatr. 2016;55:260–7.
13. Ciuffreda KJ, Kapoor N, Rutner D, Suchoff IB, Han ME, Craig S. Occurrence of oculomotor dysfunctions in acquired brain injury: a retrospective analysis. Optometry. 2007;78:155–61.
14. Hunt AW, Mah K, Reed N, Engel L, Keightley M. Oculomotor-based vision assessment in mild traumatic brain injury: a systematic review. J Head Trauma Rehabil. 2016;31:252–61.
15. Armstrong RA. Visual problems associated with traumatic brain injury. Clin Exp Optom. 2018;101:716–26.
16. Petit L, Tzourio N, Orssaud C, Pietrzyk U, Berthoz A, Mazoyer B. Functional neuroanatomy of the human visual fixation system. Eur J Neurosci. 1995;7:169–74.
17. Falck-Ytter T, Pettersson E, Bölte S, D'Onofrio B, Lichtenstein P, Kennedy DP. Difficulties maintaining prolonged fixation and attention-deficit/hyperactivity symptoms share genetic influences in childhood. Psychiatry Res. 2020;293:113384.
18. Ko HK, Poletti M, Rucci M. Microsaccades precisely relocate gaze in a high visual acuity task. Nat Neurosci. 2010;13:1549–53.
19. Gallaway M, Scheiman M, Mitchell GL. Vision therapy for post-concussion vision disorders. Optom Vis Sci. 2017;94:68–73.
20. Raghuram A, Cotter SA, Gowrisankaran S, et al. Postconcussion: receded near point of convergence is not diagnostic of convergence insufficiency. Am J Ophthalmol. 2019;206:235–44.
21. Faucher C, De Guise D. Spasm of the near reflex triggered by disruption of normal binocular vision. Optom Vis Sci. 2004;81:178–81.
22. Chan RV, Trobe JD. Spasm of accommodation associated with closed head trauma. J Neuroophthalmol. 2002;22:15–7.
23. Scheiman M, Grady MF, Jenewein E, et al. Frequency of oculomotor disorders in adolescents 11 to 17 years of age with concussion, 4 to 12 weeks post injury. Vis Res. 2021;183:73–80.
24. Brahm KD, Wilgenburg HM, Kirby J, Ingalla S, Chang CY, Goodrich GL. Visual impairment and dysfunction in combat-injured servicemembers with traumatic brain injury. Optom Vis Sci. 2009;86:817–25.
25. Storey EP, Master SR, Lockyer JE, Podolak OE, Grady MF, Master CL. Near point of convergence after concussion in children. Optom Vis Sci. 2017;94:96–100.
26. Santo AL, Race ML, Teel EF. Near point of convergence deficits and treatment following concussion: a systematic review. J Sport Rehabil. 2020;29:1179–93.
27. DuPrey KM, Webner D, Lyons A, Kucuk CH, Ellis JT, Cronholm PF. Convergence insufficiency identifies athletes at risk of prolonged recovery from sport-related concussion. Am J Sports Med. 2017;45:2388–93.
28. Adler PM, Cregg M, Viollier AJ, Margaret Woodhouse J. Influence of target type and RAF rule on the measurement of near point of convergence. Ophthalmic Physiol Opt. 2007;27:22–30.

29. Bevilacqua ZW, Kawata K. Procedural shortcomings with near point of convergence assessment may Lead to inappropriate prognosis of concussion injury in athletes: letter to the editor. Am J Sports Med. 2018;46:Np64–np66.
30. Alnawmasi MM, Khuu SK. Deficits in multiple object-tracking and visual attention following mild traumatic brain injury. Sci Rep. 2022;12:13727.
31. Dhawan PS, Leong D, Tapsell L, et al. King-Devick test identifies real-time concussion and asymptomatic concussion in youth athletes. Neurol Clin Pract. 2017;7:464–73.
32. Hunfalvay M, Murray NP, Mani R, Carrick FR. Smooth pursuit eye movements as a biomarker for mild concussion within 7-days of injury. Brain Inj. 2021;35:1682–9.
33. Bogle JM. Vestibular and balance dysfunction following sport-related concussion. Perspectives. 2019;4:1349–63.
34. Mucha A, Collins MW, Elbin RJ, et al. A brief Vestibular/Ocular Motor Screening (VOMS) assessment to evaluate concussions: preliminary findings. Am J Sports Med. 2014;42:2479–86.
35. Gaur S, Awasthi SK, Bhadouriya SK, Saxena R, Pathak VK, Bisht M. Efficacy of Epley's maneuver in treating BPPV patients: a prospective observational study. Int J Otolaryngol. 2015;2015:487160.
36. Rowe FJ, Hanna K, Evans JR, et al. Interventions for eye movement disorders due to acquired brain injury. Cochrane Database Syst Rev. 2018;3:Cd011290.
37. American Academy of Ophthalmology. Vision and concussion: symptoms, signs, evaluation, and treatment. Pediatrics. 2022;150(2):e2021056047.
38. Yap TP, Luu CD, Suttle CM, Chia A, Boon MY. Electrophysiological and psychophysical studies of meridional anisotropies in children with and without astigmatism. Invest Ophthalmol Vis Sci. 2019;60(6):1906–13.
39. Yap TP. Dyslexia and Vision–A review of current evidence and clinical interventions. Singapore: Medical Grapevine, 2013; pp.10–15.
40. Roper-Hall G. Historical vignette: Louis Émile Javal (1839–1907): the father of orthoptics. Am Orthopt J. 2006;57:131–6.
41. Ciuffreda KJ, Rutner D, Kapoor N, Suchoff IB, Craig S, Han ME. Vision therapy for oculomotor dysfunctions in acquired brain injury: a retrospective analysis. Optometry. 2008 Jan;79(1):18–22.
42. Applied concepts in vision therapy 2.0. Optometric Clinical Practice. 2022. Available through the Optometric Extension Program Foundation (www.oepf.org/product/applied-concepts-in-vision-therapy-2-0/). The book outlines practical guidelines on how to apply theoretical concepts into clinical practice. Section 2 includes diagnostic and therapeutic guidelines for traumatic brain injury.

Advances in Color Vision Testing

Sara I. Shoushtari and Rohan Bir Singh

1 Introduction

Alterations in color vision have been recognized for almost three centuries, and since their discovery, there have been attempts to qualify and quantify changes in color vision perception. The theory of color vision deficiency (CVD) was first proposed by John Dalton in the late eighteenth century, and reflected the recent discovery of red, green, and blue as primary colors [1, 2]. The earliest tests of color vision were developed to test vocational capacity in transportation careers [1]. Eventually, as understanding of the perceptual changes present in CVD grew, tests were designed to leverage the unique physiology of color vision for determination of perceptual deficiencies.

In this chapter, we will review the basic mechanisms of color perception, the deviations which cause CVD, and the traditional as well as the newer testing modalities for screening, diagnosing, and evaluating color perception.

2 Color Vision

2.1 Physiology of Color Vision

Vision is processed in the retina, and cone type photoreceptor cells are responsible for color vision perception. Cones contain photopigments, comprised of an opsin molecule and a retinol derivative [3, 4], which are capable of activating signaling cascades upon reaction with photons. To be able to perceive complex color patterns,

S. I. Shoushtari · R. B. Singh (✉)
Laboratory of Ocular Immunology, Transplantation, and Regeneration, Schepens Eye Research Institute, Massachusetts Eye and Ear Institute, Boston, MA, USA
e-mail: sara.shoushtari@meei.harvard.edu; rohan_singh@meei.harvard.edu

D. Shu et al. (eds.), *Current Advances in Optometry*, Current Practices in Ophthalmology, https://doi.org/10.1007/978-981-97-8140-9_6

the retina employs three cone types, that when combined, include most of the UV light spectrum. Short (peak sensitivity ~419 nm), medium (peak sensitivity ~530 nm), and long (peak sensitivity ~560 nm) wavelength cones correspond to blue, green, and red wavelengths, respectively. Activation of cone photopigments therefore depends on the UV wavelength of the source. The relative signaling pattern of cones is interpreted by the brain to form color vision perception.

2.2 Color Vision Deficiency

CVD has traditionally been considered a congenital disease caused by alteration or absence in one or more cone types. More commonly though, CVD occurs due to retinal or optic nerve damage from chronic disease or ocular toxic medications, leading to acquired changes in color vision, which do not usually result in chromatic patterns of loss as seen in inherited CVD.

2.2.1 Congenital Color Vision Deficiency

Congenital CVD arises from dysfunction or nonfunctional photopigments, resulting in changes or limitations in the perceived color spectrum. The prefixes protan-, deutran-, and tritan, refer to red, green, and blue, respectively, and are used when describing CVD type (Fig. 1).

Dysfunction without complete loss of photopigment causes anomalous trichromacy, and individuals will demonstrate altered hue matching patterns [3–5]. Depending on the affected cone type, individuals can be described as protanomalous, deuteranomalous, or tritanomalous. In the cause of protanomaly and deuteranomaly, individuals inherit defective long and medium wavelength sensitive photopigments with altered lengths of peak sensitivity [4]. Mutations in the short wavelength sensitivity photopigment result in tritanomaly [6].

Dichromatic vision is similarly chromatically categorized, and results from complete absence of one photopigment type, with possible associated loss in cone type within the retinal cell population [7, 8].

Monochromatism is extremely rare and results in achromatopsia, complete loss of color discrimination. Rod monochromatism is the most severe form and is due to an autosomal recessive mutation causing total absence of cone function [9]. The more common form of monochromatism is X-linked recessive blue monochromatism, where individuals only possess blue pigment cones [10]. Vision is mostly reliant on rods in blue monochromats, therefore resulting in decreased overall visual acuity.

"Red-green color-blindness" is the most common X-linked recessive vision deficiency, and includes protanomaly, deuteranomaly, protanopia, and deuteranopia, of which deuteranomaly is the most common deficiency [3]. Red-green color deficiency has a global prevalence estimated to between 2–8% in males and 0.5% in females [3]. Comparatively, "blue-yellow color blindness" consists of the "tritan deficiencies" tritanopia and tritanomaly. Tritanopia has an autosomal dominant inheritance pattern with an estimated 1 in 500 prevalence [3, 4, 6].

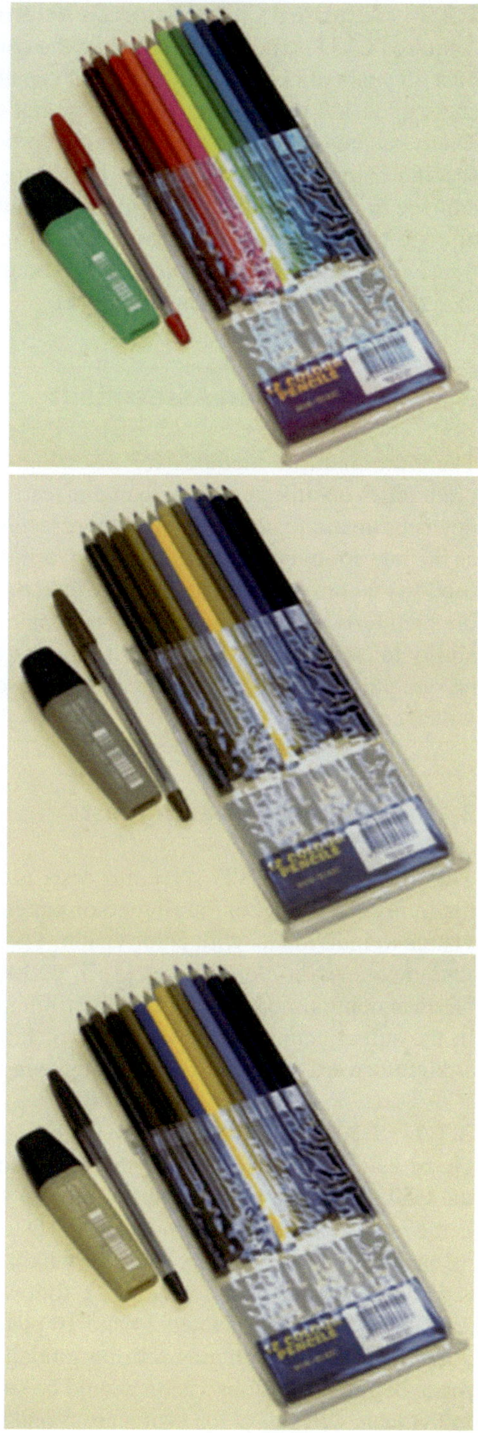

Fig. 1 Normal color vision (top) as compared to deuteranopic (middle) and proanopic (bottom) vision

2.2.2 Acquired Color Vision Deficiency

Acquired CVD is more common than the congenital form, especially in individuals over 40 years old [11]. Acquired CVD can also be associated with changes in other areas of visual perception, such as spatial discrimination and visual acuity [12]. There is some evidence of a relationship between visual perception changes and specific color deficiency patterns [12]. Most forms of acquired CVD result from damage to the retina or optic nerve, and thus there is no distinct chromatic pattern of cone loss as seen in congenital CVD [5]. Additionally, there are some medications with a known side effect of dyschromatopsia, many with unclear mechanisms of acting on the color vision system [5].

3 Color Vision Assessment

There are multiple methods for assessing CVD, and thorough clinical evaluation often relies on utilizing more than one test. The most recognized test uses the pseudoisochromatic plates (PIP) used in screening for CVD. More complex tests, such as the hue arrangement testing (Farnsworth D15) and anomaloscope evaluation, are used to diagnose specific deficiency patterns. There are also several occupationally oriented tests used by various professional institutions to determine an individual's ability to complete work specific tasks. Importantly, all testing methods utilize the unique physiology of color perception to isolate and evaluate the function of individual cone types.

3.1 Routine Screening Tests

The basis of most CVD screening tests is the PIP. PIP tests are made by placing randomly sized dots of varying color patterns to draw out numbers or shapes only visible to individuals with color vision. The variations of the color patterns can differentiate specific deficiencies [1, 3, 4, 13]. The first PIP test was developed by German ophthalmologist, Dr. Jakob Stilling in the late nineteenth century [1, 4], and in the subsequent century variations of these original tests have been made. The straightforward nature of CVD testing using PIPs makes them ideal for screening.

3.1.1 Ishihara Plates

Dr. Ishihara first published his "tests for color blindness" in 1917, where he debuted the Ishihara plates, his adaption of Stilling's PIP [14]. Today, the Ishihara plate test is the most commonly administered CVD test. The original Ishihara test consists of 38 plates, one introductory plate in which the pattern is visible to all individuals regardless of cone function (Fig. 2), following by a series of testing plates [4, 13, 15]. Subsequent abbreviated 24 and 16 plate versions have also been published [4, 13]. Each version contains scoring guideline indicating how many errors can be made before anomalous vision should be suspected [4]. This is important to note as individuals will full color vision are prone to errors when tested [16]. The Ishihara

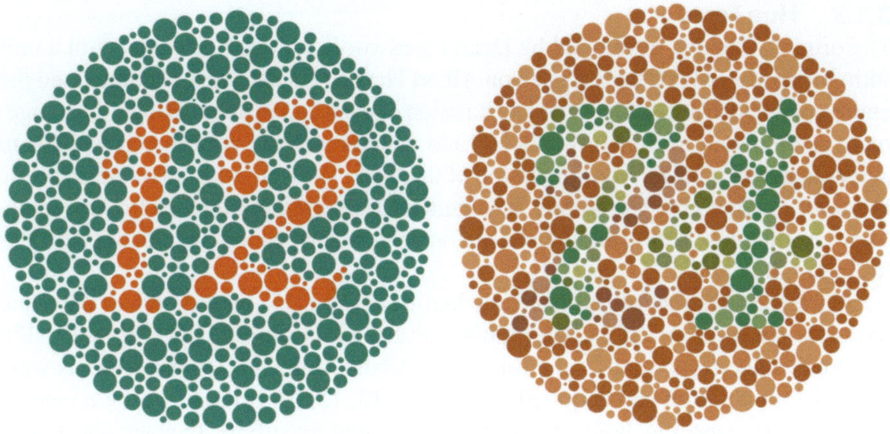

Fig. 2 Ishihara plate #1 (left), the test plate, would show "12" in all individuals regardless of color vision. Ishihara plate #9 (right) which would show "74" for normal trichromats and "21" for dichromats

plates are considered reliable screening tests for congenital red-green deficiency, with over 95% sensitivity and almost 100% specificity [17–19]. Ishihara plates are unable to determine severity of deficiency though [1, 13, 20]. Additionally, the Ishihara plates do not contain tritan sensitive plates, and therefore cannot be used to detect tritan deficiency [1, 4].

3.1.2 Hardy-Rand-Rittler (HRR) Plates

The HRR plates employ pseudoisochromatic theory to test both red-green and blue color vision deficiency, and have the ability indicate potential severity of CVD. HRR plates utilize changes in saturation of figure dots as compared to background dots to determine mild, moderate, or severe deficiency [1, 4, 13, 15, 21]. Additionally, HRR plate figures are symbols, rather than numerals, making it capable of testing younger children or those without education [1]. HRR plates are equally sensitive (1.0) and specific (over 0.97) in determining CVD [19, 21, 22].

Additional variations of PIP tests have been developed throughout the years in attempt to address the diagnostic shortcomings of the Ishihara tests and better evaluate tritan deficient and illiterate individuals [23].

Diagnostic Tests

Diagnostic tests have been developed for administration following screening tests to further classify the deficiency present. Because of this, they are inclusive of all color deficiencies, acquired and congenital, across the chromatic spectrum [1]. The most common diagnostic test is a form of an arrangement test, in which an individual arranges small caps filled with hues into their perceived natural order. The subjective order is then plotted to determine the specific CVD [4]. Variations of the tests allow for more sophisticated determination of deficiency as well as recognition of acquired variances.

3.1.3 Hue Tests

The original hue test developed by Dean Farnsworth included 100 caps with a uniform increase between hues (based on Albert Henry Munsell) that encompassed the entire color spectrum [1, 24–26]. The location of each cap in an individual's arrangement is compared to the correct order, and deviation in the pattern corresponds to perceptual deficiencies. Administration of the F-M D100 and scoring of the response is a very tedious process, so hue arrangement tests are not suitable for screening. They can diagnose subtle anomalous vision changes that cannot be identified on PIP testing [4, 22].

Shortened versions of the hue test, like the F-M D15, include fewer caps and therefore are more useful in determining severe and acquired CVD [1, 4, 13, 27]. Alternative hue tests, such as the Lanthony, Adams, and City University tests were designed for children and acquired CVD [1, 4, 13, 15, 27–30]. Hue test are considered extremely specific, however due to their limited sensitivity, they are considered more effective as follow-up tests to PIP screening [17, 19, 31].

Online hues tests are also available such as, https://www.color-blind-test.com/d15-color-blind-test-more, https://www.color-blindness.com/color-arrangement-test/. The online test consists of 15 color squares and one reference color square (Fig. 3). The patients are asked to be seated at 50 cm from computer monitor as then it subtends an angle of 1.5°. The patients begin with the reference color and arrange the others in a progression of hue and 2 minutes are given to complete the test. They are allowed to review their ordering and make any necessary changes.

For scoring, color difference vector (CVD) analysis is done. Quantifiable square arrangements include the confusion angle, which identifies the type of color vision deficiency. An angle above +0.7 degrees points toward a protan defect, between +0.7 and −65 a deutan defect and below that a tritan defect. Other parameters include the major and minor radius which is ratio of those two numbers results in the S-index. The total error score (TES) which combines the two radii into a score of total error. TES ranges from around 11 up to about 40 for strong vision deficiencies. The confusion index (C-index) quantifies the ratio between major radius and the major radius of a perfect arrangement. People with normal color vision or slightly colorblind persons have a ratio below 1.2. The higher this number (grows up to above a ratio of 4), the more is severity of color blindness.

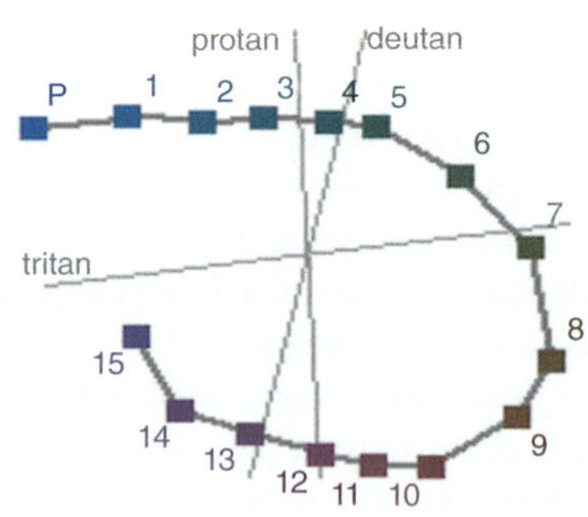

Fig. 3 Output of an online hue test (https://www.color-blindness.com/color-arrangement-test/). (Image courtesy: Dr. Parul Ichhpujani)

3.1.4 Anomaloscope

The anomaloscope is considered the gold standard of CVD diagnostic testing. An anomaloscope is an instrument to test color matching. An individual mixes two light beams to adjust the proportion of each light until they feel it matches a given sample [4, 15, 32, 33].

The results of the test are interpreted using various equations to assess the degree and type of color deficiency. The original anomaloscope was created for evaluation of red-green color deficiency using the Rayleigh equation, which dictates the tests wavelength parameters [4, 32]. The Moreland test was subsequently created to allowing for tritan deficiency testing, and similarly provides parameters and evaluation criteria [32, 34]. Alternative versions, such as the Pickford-Lakowski or Besancon test similarly can be used to assess tritan deficiency [4].

As every color on a computer display is essentially made from the base colors red, green, and blue, an anomaloscope cannot be reproduced online. Therefore, a simplistic reproduction, based on a different operating principle has been attempted on portals such as, www.color-blind-test.com/anomaloscope-more.html.

3.2 Occupational Testing

The origins of CVD tests are in occupational testing, and the first standardized color vision tests were developed to assess rail and naval employees' abilities to safely complete work duties [4]. Today various professional organizations continue to include CVD testing in employee assessments to determine the ability of an individual to perform occupational tasks [10, 31, 35].

3.2.1 Lantern

The most common occupational test in use dates to the nineteenth century, developed in response to repeated railway accidents at the time [4]. Lantern tests involve showing various color signals and patterns to individuals and asking them to state what they have been presented. The colors, speed, and spatial patterns of the test should reflect relevant occupational distinction requirements and mimic real signals the individuals would encounter [4, 27]. Thus, the lantern tests are not reliable for screening or diagnosis of CVD and should only be used to determine potentially hazardous visual defects [1, 4].Additionally, performance on lantern test cannot be easily associated with performance on other CVD tests and accordingly should not be used as a means of independent clinical diagnosis of CVD [13, 36, 37].

3.3 New Testing Modalities

With the development of technology and understanding of color perception, new testing modalities have been developed to attempt to improve the CVD screening and diagnosis process.

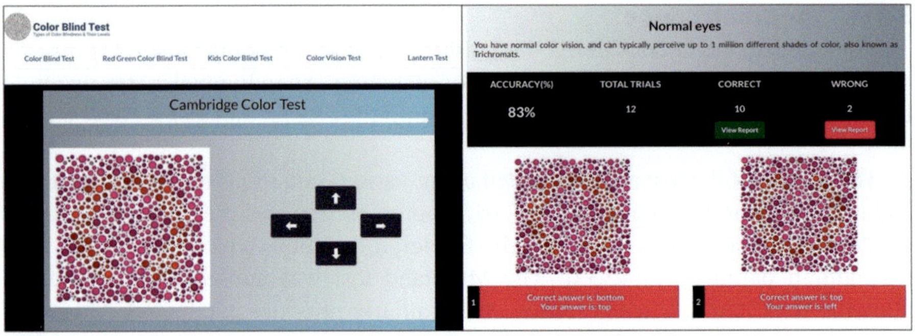

Fig. 4 Author's own test taken online, https://colorblind-test.io/cambridge-color-test

3.3.1 Digital Testing

The major innovation in CVD testing has been in the creation of various digital tests with the goal of standardizing test administration and results. Examples of digital tests include the Cambridge color test (CCT), the portal color sort test (PCST), color assessment and Diagnosis (CAD) test, and Martin Lantern test [15, 19, 27, 35, 38].

The CCT is an adaptive digital PIP test that randomizes plate order as individuals answer (Fig. 4) [15, 27]. The CCT can also be adapted for use with children, further expanding its accessibility for CVD screening [39]. The PCST offers a digital version of the hue arrangement test that allows for both screening and diagnosis [38]. The CAD test utilizes HRR plate style coloring to detect red-green deficiency [19]. Digital lantern tests, such as the Martin Lantern test, have also been developed to more easily test potential job candidates [27]. These digital tests demonstrate similar reliability to physical tests [17, 19, 31, 38].

3.3.2 Developments to PIP

Physical PIP tests also remain useful, and there have been developments in plate design to reduce variability and deterioration of plates overtime. Dalton's PIP utilizes polymer print, rather than ink to produce hues, reducing the effects of aging on testing reliability [40].

3.3.3 Electroretinography

Electroretinography (ERG) utilizes measurements of electrical signaling in the retina in response to light flashes to determine anomalies in color vision [27, 41]. ERG offers an opportunity to further objectify CVD testing and decrease reliance on subjective response to visual prompts for diagnosis [42, 43].

4 Limitations of Testing

The sensitivity and specificity of various CVD tests have been evaluated numerous times and are extremely high across testing modalities and subsequent test versions [13, 17–19, 21, 22, 31, 32, 40, 44]. However, there remains several limitations to the currently available CVD testing methods.

The most common issue with physically administered tests is the possibility for variation. This can be a result of differences in ambient lighting during testing or hue quality on plates and caps. Tests contain instructions on standard lighting conditions to effectively administer the test [4]. There have been several studies that demonstrate that changes in lighting source during testing can either improve anomalous performance or increase failures in trichromats [45–50]. Additionally, physical plates and hue caps have the potential to deteriorate over time, also affecting performance of both normal and anomalous individuals. However, these limitations can also apply to digital test, which must be similarly standardized to reduce the effect of display screen variance on test efficacy [27].

Another limitation of current CVD testing methods is the lack of standardization across tests [15]. Scores between modalities are not comparable and therefore grading of CVD severity is not uniform. Furthermore, there is no current procedure for testing that allows for complete screening and diagnosis within one test. It is frequently recommended that more than one test be utilized to ensure diagnose [4, 15].

A concern for many institutions that administer tests for occupational evaluation is attempts to memorize test to ensure passing despite CVD [31]. This is especially common with plate and lantern tests that have limited ability to randomize or adapt to individual responses [31]. Digital tests that adapt to individual response, or more complex tests such as hue arrangement, can provide a more reliable assessment of color vision [15, 27, 38].

Improvement has been made to make CVD screening more accessible to individuals with intellectual disability, poor literacy, and children, however, many tests remain inaccessible. Hue sorting test require physical mobility, and many PIP tests require recognition of numerals [4].

5 Future Directions

Augmented reality and virtual reality technologies are being explored to create immersive color vision testing environments. These platforms offer novel ways to simulate real-world color discrimination tasks and evaluate color vision under various lighting conditions, potentially improving the ecological validity of assessments.

Machine learning algorithms and AI techniques are being applied to analyze large datasets of color vision test results [51]. These approaches can identify patterns and correlations that may not be apparent to human observers, potentially leading to new insights into color vision disorders and more accurate diagnostic algorithms.

6 Conclusion

Color vision deficiency testing utilizes the unique physiology of human color perception to isolate the function of cone types and assess their function and the principles of color vision testing have remained the same for centuries. Developments have been made recently to improve test administration and increase test accessibility, however, many issues with standardized test experiences remain. Progress also needs to be made to create tests that are better able to screen, diagnose, and offer useful evaluation of an individual's functional and occupational ability. As our understanding of retinal cell development increases, there will be great opportunities to apply this knowledge to better understand color vision and offer new methods for testing and predicting CVD.

References

1. French A, Rose K, Thompson K, Cornell E. The evolution of colour vision testing. Aust Orthopt J. 2008;40:7–15.
2. Dalton J. Extraordinary facts relating to the vision of colours: with observations. England-Manchester: Cadell and Davies; 1794.
3. Simunovic MP. Colour vision deficiency. Eye (Lond). 2010;24:747–55.
4. Melamud A, Hagstrom S, Traboulsi EI. Color vision testing. Ophthalmic Genet. 2004;25:159–87.
5. Simunovic MP. Major review acquired color vision deficiency. Surv Ophthalmol. 2016;61:132–55.
6. Weitz CJ, Went LN, Nathans J. Human tritanopia associated with a third amino acid substitution in the blue-sensitive visual pigment. Am J Hum Genet. 1992;51:444–6.
7. Baraas RC, Carroll J, Gunther KL, Chung M, Williams DR, Foster DH, Neitz M. Adaptive optics retinal imaging reveals S-cone dystrophy in Tritan color-vision deficiency. J Opt Soc Am. 2007;24:1438–47.
8. Carroll J, Neitz M, Hofer H, Neitz J, Williams DR, Nathans J. Functional photoreceptor loss revealed with adaptive optics: an alternate cause of color blindness. Proc Natl Acad Sci USA. 2004;101:8461–6.
9. Kohl S, Marx T, Giddings I, Jägle H, Jacobson SG, Apfelstedt-Sylla E, Zrenner E, Sharpe LT, Wissinger B. Total colourblindness is caused by mutations in the gene encoding the α-subunit of the cone photoreceptor CGMP-gated cation channel. Nat Genet. 1998;19:257–9.
10. Nathans J, Davenport CM, Maumenee IH, Lewis RA, Fielding Hejtmancik J, Litt M, Lovrien E, Weleber R, Bachynski B, Zwas F, et al. Molecular genetics of human blue cone monochromacy. Science. 1989;245:831–8.
11. Schneck ME, Haegerstrom-Portnoy G, Lott LA, Brabyn JA. Comparison of Panel D-15 Tests in a large older population. Optom Vis Sci. 2014;91:284–90.
12. Verriest G. Further studies on acquired deficiency of color discrimination. J Opt Soc Am. 1963;53:185–95.
13. Cole BL. Assessment of inherited colour vision defects in clinical practice. Clin Exp Optom. 2007;90:157–75.
14. Ishihara S. Tests for colour-blindness. Tokyo: Handaya Hongo Harukich; 1917.
15. Zarazaga AF, Gutiérrez Vásquez J, Royo VP. Revisión de Los Principales Test Clínicos Para Evaluar La Del Color. Arch Soc Esp Oftalmol. 2019;94:25–32.
16. Miyahara E. Errors reading the Ishihara pseudoisochromatic plates made by observers with normal colour vision. Clin Exp Optom. 2008;91:161–5.
17. Marechal M, Delbarre M, Tesson J, Lacambre C, Lefebvre H, Froussart-Maille F. Color vision tests in pilots' medical assessments. Aerosp Med Hum Perform. 2018;89:737–43.
18. Birch J. Efficiency of the Ishihara Test for identifying red-green colour deficiency. Ophthalmic Physiol Opt. 1997;17:403–8.
19. Seshadri J, Christensen J, Bassi CJ. Evaluation of the new web-based "Colour Assessment and Diagnosis" Test. Optom Vis Sci. 2005;82:882–5.
20. Hardy H, Rand G, Rittler MC. Tests for detection and analysis of color blindness: an evaluation of the Ishihara Test. Arch Ophthalmol. 1945;34:295–302.

21. Cole BL, Lian KY, Lakkis C. The new Richmond HRR Pseudoisochromatic Test for colour vision is better than the Ishihara Test. Clin Exp Optom. 2006;89:73–80.
22. Birch J. Clinical use of the American Optical Company (Hardy, Rand and Rittler) pseudoisochromatic plates for red-green colour deficiency. Ophthal Physiol Opt. 1997;17:248–54.
23. Alduhayan R, Almustanyir A. Comparison of two printed pseudoisochromatic tests for color vision assessment. Optom Vis Sci. 2023;100(12):840–6.
24. Farnsworth D. The Farnsworth-Munsell 100-Hue and Dichotomous Tests for color vision*. JOSA. 1943;33:568–78.
25. Munsell AH. A color notation: a measured color system based on the three qualities, Hue, Values and Chroma with illustrative models, charts and a course of study arranged for teachers. Boston: Geo H Ellis Co; 1907.
26. Hasrod N, Rubin A. Colour vision: a review of the Cambridge Colour Test and other colour testing methods. Afr Vision Eye Health. 2015;74:23.
27. Lanthony P. The desaturated Panel D-15. Doc Ophthalmol. 1978;46:185–9.
28. Dain SJ, Adams AJ. Comparison of the Standard and Adams Desaturated D-15 Tests with congenital colour vision deficiencies. Ophthalmic Physiol Opt. 1990;10:40–5.
29. Birch J. Clinical use of the City University Test (2nd Edition). Ophthalmic Physiol Opt. 1997;17:466–72.
30. Walsh DV, Robinson J, Jurek GM, Capó-Aponte JE, Riggs DW, Temme LA. A performance comparison of color vision tests for military screening. Aerosp Med Hum Perform. 2016;87:382–7.
31. Zabel J, Przekoracka-Krawczyk A, Olszewski J, Michalak KP. Variability of Rayleigh and Moreland Test results using anomaloscope in young adults without color vision disorders. PLoS One. 2021;16:e0251903.
32. Nagel WA. Zwei Apparate Für Die Augenärztliche Funktionsprüfung Adaptometer Und Kleines Spektralphotometer (Anomaloskop). Zeitschrift für Augenheilkunde. 1907;17:201–22.
33. Pokorny J, Smith VC, Went LN. Color matching in autosomal dominant Tritan defect. J Opt Soc Am. 1981;71:1327.
34. Gao H, Kirkendall CD, Kinney MJ, Preston AM, Reddix MD. Color vision testing, standards, and visual performance of the U.S. Military. Mil Med. 2023;188:49–57.
35. Cole B, Maddocks J. Can clinical colour vision test be used to predict the Farnsworth Lantern Test? Vis Res. 1998;38:3483–5.
36. Birch J. Performance of colour-deficient people on the Holmes-Wright Lantern (Type A): consistency of occupational colour vision standards in aviation. Ophthalmic Physiol Opt. 2008;28:253–8.
37. Melamud A, Simpson E, Traboulsi EI. Introducing a new computer-based test for the clinical evaluation of color discrimination. Am J Ophthalmol. 2006;142:953–60.
38. Goulart PRK, Bandeira ML, Tsubota D, Oiwa NN, Costa MF, Ventura DF. A computer-controlled color vision test for children based on the Cambridge Colour Test. Vis Neurosci. 2008;25:445–50.
39. Narayanan A, Venkadesan M, Krishnamurthy SS, Hussaindeen JR, Ramani KK. Dalton's pseudo-isochromatic plates and congenital colour vision deficiency. Clin Exp Optom. 2020;103:853–7.
40. Crognale MA, Teller DY, Motulsky AG, Deeb SS. Severity of color vision defects: electroretinographic (ERG): molecular and behavioral studies. Vis Res. 1998;38:3377–85.
41. Aher AJ, Martins CMG, Barboni MTS, Nagy BV, Hauzman E, Bonci DMO, Ventura DF, Kremers J. Electroretinographical determination of human color vision type. J Opt Soc Am A. 2018;35:B92.
42. Hovis JK, Leat SJ, Heffernan S, Epp K. The validity of the University of Waterloo Colored Dot Test for color vision testing in adults and preschool children. Optom Vis Sci. 2002;79:241–53.
43. Schmidt I. Effect of illumination in testing color vision with pseudo-isochromatic plates. J Opt Soc Am. 1952;42:951–5.

44. Zahiruddin K, Banu S, Dharmarajan R, Kulothungan V, Vijayan D, Raman R, Sharma T. Effect of illumination on colour vision testing with Farnsworth-Munsell 100 Hue Test: customized colour vision booth versus room illumination. Korean J Ophthalmol. 2010;24:159–62.
45. Wall M, Donzis PB, Wall MM. Luminance contrast and colour contrast related errors in pseudoisochromatic plate identification. Eye. 1997;11:713–6.
46. Tamura S, Okamoto Y, Nakagawa S, Sakamoto T, Ando M, Shigeri Y. Light wavelengths of LEDs to improve the color discrimination in Ishihara Test and Farnsworth Panel D-15 Test for Deutans. Color Res Appl. 2017;42:424–30.
47. Hardy LH, Rand G, Catherine Rittler M, New YA. Effect of quality of illumination on the results of the Ishihara Test. J Opt Soc Am. 1946;6:86–94.
48. Katavisto M. Pseudo-isochromatic plates and artificial light: comparative studies of Boström's II, Ishihara's and Stilling's plates by the daylight, tungsten lamps, and fluorescent tubes. Acta Ophthalmol. 1961;39:377–90.
49. Hyon JY, Lee JH, Wee WR. Shift of colorimetric values in Ishihara pseudoisochromatic plates with plate aging. Korean J Ophthalmol. 2005;19:145–8.
50. Lee DY, Honson M. Chromatic variation of Ishihara diagnostic plates. Color Res Appl. 2003;28:267–76.
51. He J, Bex PJ, Skerswetat J. Rapid measurement and machine learning classification of colour vision deficiency. Ophthalmic Physiol Opt. 2023;43(6):1379–90.

Advances in Low Vision Aids

Samira Mortazavi and Asha Meloottu

1 Introduction

An article published in 1964 by optometrist Dr. John Zettel discusses official terminology for patients with partial vision loss, determining a need for classifying the degree of blindness due to changes in social standards at the time. Visually impaired patients were initially labeled as people with "*subnormal vision,*" however, Zettel recommended using the term "*partially sighted individuals.*" He also made an outline of recommendations for these patients, including examination techniques and low vision aids to prescribe [1].These aids included high add power bifocals and base out prism glasses with increased power to aid in convergence and fusion [1]. Today, "*visually impaired*" is the accepted terminology for this population, and the specialty in caring for these individuals can be referred to as low vision or vision rehabilitation. While high-power lenses are still widely prescribed, updated technology has diversified and increased clinicians' options in prescription low vision aids.

The goal of low vision devices is to augment or maximize the remaining vision that the patient has. When weighing appropriate devices for low vision patients, it is necessary to consider their level of visual function, the type of vision loss, the patient's cognitive function, and the visual goal they are trying to accomplish. Additionally, this decision-making process must consider the principle of least effort, where options that are easier to implement and require less labor are more favorable. Therefore, to prevent device abandonment and unnecessary patient costs, a stepwise approach is necessary for choosing low vision devices.

S. Mortazavi (✉) · A. Meloottu
Massachusetts Eye and Ear, Harvard Medical School, Boston, MA, USA
e-mail: smortazavi@mgh.harvard.edu; ameloottu@mgh.harvard.edu

D. Shu et al. (eds.), *Current Advances in Optometry*, Current Practices in Ophthalmology, https://doi.org/10.1007/978-981-97-8140-9_7

2 Low Vision Devices

Below are the general categories of devices used in low vision rehabilitation, listed in increasing complexity.

- Spectacle correction
  - High reading adds
  - Microscopes
- Magnifiers
  - Handheld magnifiers
  - Stand magnifiers
- Telescopes
  - Handheld telescopes (Galilean, Keplerian)
  - Spectacle mounted (binocular vs. monocular)
- Electronic devices
  - Desktop CCTV (with or without OCR)
  - Portable CCTV
  - Head-mounted
  - Applications for smartphones/tablets
- Non-optical devices
  - Optical Character Recognition (OCR)
  - Tactile (e.g., Braille)
  - Audio devices (e.g., Talking watches, Siri, etc.)

2.1 Devices for Mild Low Vision

These patients will fall into the visual acuity range of 20/20–20/70 (Table 1) and will easily find improvement to their visual impairments through simple optical devices. These include:

- Spectacle or contact lens correction
- High reading adds
- Microscopes
- Magnifiers
- Telescopes

Table 1 Grading of Visual Impairment [2]

Category	Worse than	Equal to or better than
Mild visual impairment		20/70
Moderate visual impairment	20/70	20/200
Severe visual impairment	20/200	20/400
Blindness	20/400	No light perception

2.2 Devices for Moderate Low Vision

These patients will fall into the visual acuity range of <20/70–20/200. The patient's overall visual function becomes dependent on how both eyes work together. For example, if the acuity of one eye still falls into the category of mild low vision, they may still benefit from simple optical devices alone. However, if vision loss is complicated by central scotomas or visual confusion the visual potential is limited and these patients may function more similarly to someone with severe low vision. In such cases, electronic devices and smartphone applications may be more efficient at improving visual function (See Sect. 2.3). Similarly, when patients have a hemianopsia following a stroke or traumatic brain injury, their visual function is greatly impeded, though central visual acuity is spared. In these scenarios, patients may benefit from a peripheral prism (ex: Peli Prisms) to expand their awareness of the missing field.

2.3 Devices for Severe Low Vision—Blindness

These patients will fall into the visual acuity range of <20/200-no light perception. At this stage, optical devices are often dependent on the acuity of both eyes individually (as stated above). Patients will likely gain some benefit from optical devices and will rely more on devices that augment their vision, such as electronic devices. When the visual impairment is very severe to total blindness, the patient must rely on other senses to function. This may mean using auditory cues from optical character recognition devices or tactile cues.

2.4 Current and Emerging Low Vision Aids

In the early 1800s, a young Louis Braille was introduced to *night writing*, a tactile writing system that uses 12 raised dots in various arrangements. While night writing was originally invented by Charles Barbier for soldiers to communicate in the dark, Braille simplified and perfected the system by reducing the 12 dots arrangements to 6 dots and changing the symbols to stand for letters rather than sounds [3]. The braille system is a well-known adaptation still used for visually impaired individuals and can be implemented presently as an accommodation. While braille is still taught to children with vision impairment, adults are encouraged toward low vision aids that can be seamlessly integrated into their life. Older individuals may not want the extensive training required to learn a new way of reading or may struggle with using tactile cues due to other comorbidities. Other available accommodations, such as magnification, do not require learning a new language and allow patients to continue enjoying reading material they are familiar with.

Magnification-Optical magnifiers such as handheld, dome, and stand magnifiers are commonly prescribed, due to being user-friendly, affordable, and often portable. Traditionally, the potential magnification to read standard size print (1M) can be determined with the patient's recorded working distance and acuity. Based on this calculation, a low vision specialist can provide the patient with a demonstration and a prescription for an optical magnifier. The magnification of a handheld or stand magnifier cannot be adjusted; therefore, if vision continues to decline, a magnifier with a lower power may be deemed useless to the patient. Video magnification, on the other hand, such as portable digital magnifiers and CCTVs (closed circuit televisions), can adjust magnification strength while providing other vision-enhancing possibilities such as adjusting contrast and brightness. Video magnifiers can offer magnification from 2× to 60×, providing patients the flexibility not offered by optical magnifiers. Another added benefit of digital magnifiers is comfort, primarily through having a larger screen and a more natural reading position. Digital and video magnifiers often include built-in stands that allow the screen to face the patient at an angle or, in the case of desktop CCTVs, straight ahead. Unlike dome and stand magnifiers, patients are not required to hover over the device to read on a flat surface.

Electronic Magnification-Currently, there is a shift toward prescribing digital magnification, such as desktop CCTVs, portable video magnifiers, and magnifying smartphone applications. As mentioned, in addition to the possibility of adjusting the magnification provided by the video magnifier, another substantial benefit of such devices is the ability to change the text's contrast. Contrast sensitivity is a measure of visual function that describes the ability to differentiate the target luminance from the background luminance [4]. This measurement can be done with a Pelli-Robson Chart or a MARS chart to find the logarithmic value of the contrast sensitivity of the patient. Different values are assigned for different age groups and are categorized as normal, moderate loss, severe loss, and profound loss. Contrast sensitivity impairment is less commonly reported than visual acuity but may better represent real-world goals and situations [4]. Visual acuity charts used in the exam room are known to have 100% contrast with black letters on a white background. However, the patient will likely encounter everyday circumstances that require high contrast sensitivity, which become more critical on cloudy days, indoors, and in other low lighting settings. A sign of reduced contrast can be difficulty seeing faces or reading a newspaper, as both have a relatively low target to background luminance ratio compared to a standard visual acuity chart. There are numerous studies regarding the decrease in contrast sensitivity for various ocular diseases, and even a study showing that glaucoma patients may have impaired contrast sensitivity while having good visual acuity [5].

There are several methods to help patients with reduced contrast sensitivity. Some digital magnifiers can increase contrast by changing the color of the reading material or object being viewed. These color combinations can include an increased contrast of white background with black writing, black background with white writing, yellow background with black writing, blue background with yellow writing, and others—up to 14 different color combinations to increase the contrast of the targeted material (e.g., See Fig. 1).

Tints-A decrease in contrast sensitivity can also be addressed with light filters or tinted lenses. A tint assessment can be an element of a low vision examination, depending on the patient's vision loss and the pathology causing the loss. For

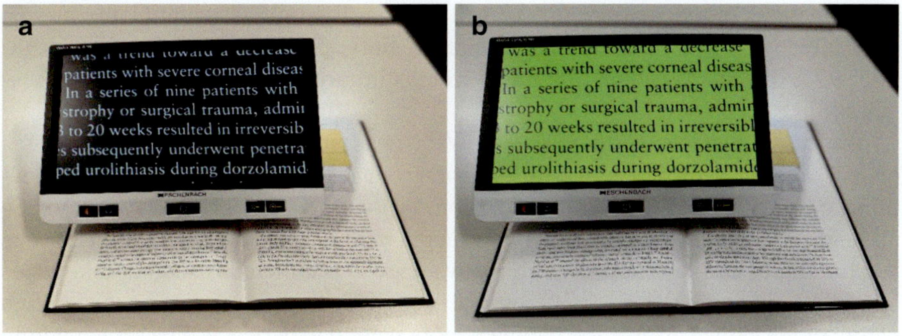

Fig. 1 (**a** and **b**) Textbook being magnified using a digital magnifier with "False Colors" setting to increase contrast

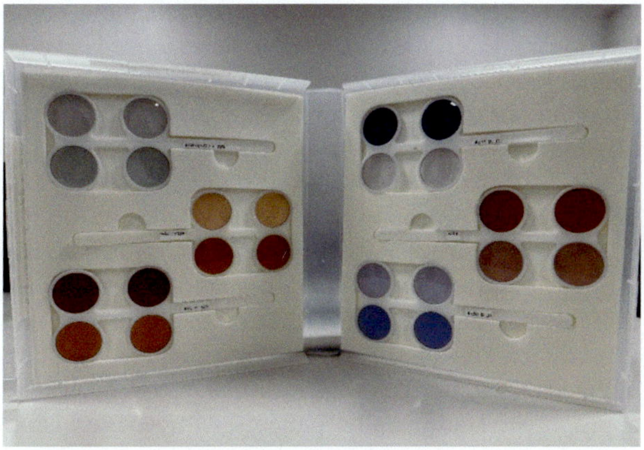

Fig. 2 Tint evaluation kit commonly used for polytrauma conditions

instance, a patient with decreased contrast sensitivity due to advanced glaucoma may express that yellow and orange tints increase contrast. This can be measured objectively by repeating contrast sensitivity testing to see if there is a notable increase in score. Tints can also be used for nontraditional vision impairment, such as traumatic brain injury or extreme photophobia. Particularly, lenses that block 480 nm wavelengths, like the rose-colored FL-41 tint, have been proven to aid migraine headaches and the photophobia caused by it. In one study, 37 individuals with chronic migraines were asked to trial seven different lens tints and choose the most comfortable ones [6]. The results showed that 71% of participants preferred FL-41 tinted lenses to aid in their migraine symptoms [6].

Tints can also be used for glare sensitivity caused by ocular pathology. In-office tint assessments can be done with tint kits (Fig. 2). These tints can be prescribed to be placed in habitual glasses or as an addition to glasses, such as a fit-over frame or a clip-on. Corning, a large glass company, introduced corning protective color filter (CPF) lenses in the 1980's, and these have been the industry standard for tinted lenses [7]. Currently, many companies offer corning *inspired* lenses, offering interpretations of the same colors as well as other light filters scientifically proven to be effective [7]. In addition to light filtering tints, glare reducing tints, like NoIR, filter 99% of short wavelength light as well as infrared light to help reduce excess glare [8].

Wearable Devices-Virtual reality (VR) headsets enable augmentation of a patient's visual acuity or expansion of their visual field through a wearable electronic device. Devices such as the IrisVision, Vision Buddy, eSight, and PatriotVision all employ a camera that feeds a video image onto the internal device screen. The head-mounted displays have a similar advantage to traditional binocular telescopes as digital magnifiers have with optical magnifiers—flexibility. The hands-free nature of the device affords the patient a more natural experience. The screen within the headset allows for variable magnification using digital zoom, contrast enhancements, and minification. While older VR devices are reportedly uncomfortable due to the weight placed on the patient's head, newer devices such as the IrisVision Inspire and eSight Go are designed to fit more ergonomically, similar to glasses [9–11]. While VR devices work for visual needs at all distances, they are more beneficial for distance viewing. Many versions include OCR (Optical Character Recognition) capabilities for reading, a live feed from the patient's cable box for TV viewing, phone connectivity for smartphone use, and voice control settings. The use of VR devices while mobile is discouraged, as proprioception changes with magnification and minification [12].

Optical Character Recognition (OCR)-Not all patients with visual impairment can read comfortably with magnification alone. If vision reduction is more severe, or scotomas and field loss interrupt the natural flow of reading, attempting to increase reading ability may be frustrating and cumbersome for the patient. In these circumstances, devices that utilize audio instead of visual support may be more appropriate. Traditionally, patients with severe vision loss were limited to prerecorded audiobooks and prerecorded object identification using barcode scanning. This restricted identification to objects that had barcodes, and often would only identify the object without providing more helpful information. For example, these devices may be able to correctly identify a can of food but not read cooking instructions written on the back. Optical character recognition, also known as text recognition, deciphers printed text and converts it to a digital format. This technology aids patients in reading virtually anything, including bills, newspapers, magazines, and even text on everyday items. Devices with OCR capabilities range from desktop CCTVs to wearable technology. Desktop devices such as Lyric or Eye-Pal Solo can be a simple option for older patients or patients who don't require the portability of alternative aids. The primary benefit of these devices is the oversized tactile buttons, which many patients find easier to utilize.

Smartphone Technology-There are many smart device applications for visually impaired individuals, such as SeeingAI, EnVision, and Lookout-Assisted Vision. These applications may be equipped with OCR technology, artificial intelligence to describe a scene, options to help patients find an object in a room, and various other features. OCR features within a smartphone application have the benefit of being an inexpensive, more simplistic, and more immediate option when compared to desktop OCR devices Smartphones also have built-in accessibility options for visually impaired individuals that can be customized in the phone's settings. Apple iPhones have features such as zoom, magnifier, audio descriptions, and dictation, to name a few [13]. Android phones are also equipped with similar accessibility options, including customizing screen contrast, "talk back" or the screen's ability to be read aloud, and text magnification [14]. Both smartphone companies have tutorials that are available for patients and family members to make these accessibility changes as an initial step toward independence with visual impairment. These accessibility options allow a more seamless transition for patients to continue using a device they are already familiar with. This also allows visually impaired individuals to not draw attention to their impairment should that be a concern to them. Clinicians should familiarize themselves with these accessibility options to help patients set up their phones for their low vision assessment in the clinic.

Similar to smartphone use described above, not all technology beneficial to visually impaired individuals was originally made for that purpose. Voice assistants such as Apple's Siri, Microsoft's Cortana, Amazon's Alexa, and Google Assistant are available on smartphones or speaker devices. Siri and Google Assistant can send and read texts, make phone calls, answer basic questions, set timers, and carry out many other commands. Individuals without vision impairment use these voice assistants regularly, but they also prove to be highly beneficial for low vision individuals. Smart home automation using Google Home and Alexa may also support low vision individuals. Installing commands such as turning lights or appliances on/off make previously difficult tasks for low vision individuals achievable with a few spoken words. The thermostat may even be set to a specific temperature, rather than manually adjusting it, negating the need for a handheld magnifier to see the small numbers.

Mobility Aids-People with vision impairment face mobility challenges with navigating indoor and outdoor settings [15]. For this specific functional challenge, white canes and seeing-eye dogs continue to be commonly used among this population. White canes provide the user beneficial feedback for obstacles in front of them to encourage more independence while ambulating. However, learning to use a white cane takes multiple training sessions from orientation and mobility specialists to ensure confidence in the user. Newer technology aims to decrease the training needed for traditional mobility aids as much as possible to encourage seamless integration in the user's life. This aspect is especially crucial for older patients whose vision loss occurs later in life. Ultrasound devices on the market, such as the Buzz clip, are designed for use with the white cane. This device uses ultrasound to detect obstacles in the user's path and alert them with vibrations. The WeWALK smart handle can attach to any long cane and provides additional mobility support, including vibration to inform the patient of low-hanging obstacles that a cane alone would miss, such as a sign or tree branch. Additionally, the patient can pair their cane to the WeWALK app on iOS or Android devices via Bluetooth to make use of its public transportation features and other audio alerts [16].

With the rise in artificial intelligence use, wearable devices to aid in mobility, such as the Biped, are entering the market for testing. The Biped is a harness worn on the shoulders and is equipped with cameras, offering audio feedback to the wearer, alerting them of any obstacles. This device advertises itself to function as a "self-driving car" but for pedestrians, offering guidance to the wearer in real time [17]. The Biped is currently being used in the USA and Europe and has plans to include GPS (Global Positioning System) capabilities in upcoming updates [17]. As mentioned earlier, these wearable devices can benefit patients because of the reduced training required to utilize these devices.

Psychology Services-It is important to note that even with the devices and accommodations available for visually impaired individuals, there is not a lack of mental health difficulties associated with the loss of sight. Blindness is reported to be one of the most feared health complications, greater than cancer or paralysis. Loss of vision may cause anxiety, worry, embarrassment, and social withdrawal due to negative self-perceptions [18]. Overall, vision loss can cause emotions similar to bereavement, due to the loss of a heavily relied-on sense. Some mental health difficulties may stem from visual hallucinations that often occur with vision loss [20]. Patients may not report these hallucinations in fear of being perceived as having a psychiatric disorder and are, therefore, less likely to receive support. In addition to having an examination with a low vision provider, it is important to inquire about the patient's adaptation to their condition and offer a supportive space to share their concerns. Providing resources available in the community, support groups, and a referral to a psychiatric provider can offer patients with tools to better navigate the emotional and social changes that accompany vision loss [17]. Currently there is limited data to support the positive effects on mental health that support groups can provide [18]. As research continues, there is a high likelihood of more data to support mental health interventions in patients with vision loss.

3 Case Scenario

A 51-year-old female presented for a low vision examination with a known history of Stargardt Disease. The patient presented to the inherited retinal disease department after 4 years with no reported change to her vision. She denied any issues with her peripheral vision or night vision. Her visual acuity was 20/500 in the right eye and 20/400 in the left eye—with a slight decrease in acuity in the right eye since last seen. A battery of testing was performed, including a Goldman Visual Field of both eyes, which revealed stable, dense central scotomas. Her last low vision evaluation was several years prior and was now being referred back to the vision rehabilitation department, as she had reported some difficulty with her activities of daily living.

As a previous patient of vision rehab services, she had received several devices prior to this visit; however, she still found herself having difficulty seeing small objects around the house. She also reported increased difficulty with reading, even while using her current devices.

The following is a review of her current devices when she presented for her low vision evaluation:

1. Prism Magnifier Reading Glasses (+10D): Used for quick reading around the house (e.g., reading labels in the kitchen), however found that this device was not enough.
2. Desktop CCTV: Working well, used mostly for reading.
3. Computer enlargement software: Used for reading emails, and other computer work - working well.
4. Ruby XL HD portable electronic magnifier: Working well, however, used infrequently as it was cumbersome to carry around the house or outside the house.
5. Smartphone accessibility settings: Patient is using all the accessibility settings on her phone without difficulty. Not using any apps for magnification.
6. Eschenbach 7× handheld optical magnifier: Uses occasionally, working fine.
7. Long cane: No difficulty, no new mobility goals.
8. Beecher 5.5× binocular telescope: Working well uses this device most frequently for distance viewing needs.
9. IrisVision head-mounted device: Using infrequently in the garden, watching TV, reading.

Her main goal with this exam was to improve reading, and so while the above devices did not adequately meet this need, the following devices were shown to her:

1. iPhone apps such as SeeingAI and Magnifier
2. +16 prism readers—custom made

3.1 Case Take Aways

- The simpler devices were what the patient tended to use more frequently (e.g., Beecher binocular telescope, prism readers), following the principle of least effort.
- Where the portable handheld CCTV (Ruby XL HD) was cumbersome to transport, smartphone applications provided similar features with the addition of other app features and ease of access (considering how consistently the patient had her phone on her person).

4 Conclusion

Low vision device technology has advanced rapidly in recent years. To keep up with the ever-increasing low vision population, it is necessary to have a good understanding of the available devices and related resources for these patients. While optical devices such as handheld magnifiers and telescopes remain within our baseline battery of low vision devices, newer technology such as VR headsets, OCR, and smartphone applications can give patients the most visual functional benefit and with the most ease. Though many devices are available for patients to use, patients are often unaware of all the tools at their disposal. Given this, it is ideal for clinicians to have a good knowledge of at least a few of these devices to better support their visually impaired patients.

References

1. Zettel J Jr. The care of low vision. Am J Optom Arch Am Acad Optom. 1964;41:142–9.
2. Tan CW. Braille and the need to innovate for the blind. Ann Acad Med Singap. 2018;47(1):1–2.
3. Paulsen AJ, Pinto A, Fischer ME, Chen Y, Huang GH, Klein BEK, Klein R, Cruickshanks KJ. Generational differences in the 10-year incidence of impaired contrast sensitivity. Ophthalmic Epidemiol. 2021;28(2):175–82.
4. Fatehi N, Nowroozizadeh S, Henry S, Coleman AL, Caprioli J, Nouri-Mahdavi K. Association of Structural and Functional Measures with contrast sensitivity in glaucoma. Am J Ophthalmol. 2017;178:129–39.
5. Reyes N, Huang JJ, Choudhury A, Pondelis N, Locatelli EVT, Hollinger R, Felix ER, Pattany PM, Galor A, Moulton EA. FL-41 tint reduces activation of neural pathways of photophobia in patients with chronic ocular pain. Am J Ophthalmol. 2024;259:172–84.
6. https://chadwickoptical.com/. Accessed 21 Jan 2024.
7. https://www.noirinsight.com/low-vision-sunglasses. Accessed 21 Jan 2024.
8. Schmidt DC, Kjølholm CDB, Torner Jordana J, Spange V, Højstrup PD, Larsen BS, Kessel L. At-home trial of four different head-mounted displays in visual rehabilitation of people with Stargardt disease. Clin Optom (Auckl). 2023;15:271–81.
9. https://irisvision.com/irisvision-inspire/. Accessed 21 Jan 2024.
10. https://www.esighteyewear.com. Accessed 21 Jan 2024.
11. Pur DR, Lee-Wing N, Bona MD. The use of augmented reality and virtual reality for visual field expansion and visual acuity improvement in low vision rehabilitation: a systematic review. Graefes Arch Clin Exp Ophthalmol. 2023;261(6):1743–55.
12. https://www.apple.com/accessibility/vision/. Accessed 21 Jan 2024.
13. https://www.android.com/accessibility/vision/. Accessed 21 Jan 2024.
14. Hoy MB. Alexa, Siri, Cortana, and more: an introduction to voice assistants. Med Ref Serv Q. 2018;37(1):81–8.
15. Access World Home, American Foundation for the blind, March 2017 https://www.afb.org/aw/18/3/15228. Accessed 21 Jan 2024.
16. https://www.biped.ai. Accessed on 21 Jan 2024.
17. Barasche-Berdah D, Paltiel O, Raz R. Active lifestyle and mobility of adults with vision impairment: a multiphase mixedmethods study. Int J Environ Res Public Health. 2023;20(19):6839.
18. Demmin DL, Silverstein SM. Visual Impairment and Mental Health: Unmet Needs and Treatment Options. Clin Ophthalmol. 2020;14:4229-51. https://doi.org/10.2147/OPTH.S258783. PMID: 33299297; PMCID: PMC7721280.

Advances in Contact Lenses for Ophthalmic Drug Delivery

Parvin Shokrollahi and Alex Hui

1 Traditional Eye Drug Dosage Forms

In contemporary practice, more than 90% of ocular drug formulations used are eye drops [1]. Despite their popularity, eye drops are generally inefficient drug delivery systems due to rapid drainage of instilled drops from the ocular surface as well as nonproductive absorption through routes leading away from the eye, resulting in short precorneal residence time and less than 5% bioavailability, respectively [1]. This inefficiency in drug delivery necessitates multiple instillations of eye drops to reach and maintain therapeutic concentrations, all of which can be significantly impacted by patient compliance. Compliance is further compounded in chronic conditions, with indefinite drug use and potential for multiple drugs being used simultaneously. Multi use formulations also contain preservatives to protect against microbial contamination but are known to have detrimental effects on the ocular surface due to their cytotoxicity [2]. Nonproductive absorption systemically can also cause detrimental side effects, with heart related complications after usage of topical beta blockers for the treatment glaucoma a ready example [3].

It is within this context that researchers have investigated other means of delivering drugs to the eye, including use of medicated or therapeutic contact lenses (TCLs). The field of drug delivery from contact lenses has seen important developments within the past decade, including the release of commercially available products. This chapter will present an overview regarding the chemistry and

P. Shokrollahi
Centre for Ocular Research and Education, University of Waterloo, Waterloo, Canada

A. Hui (✉)
School of Optometry and Vision Science, UNSW Sydney, Sydney, Australia
e-mail: alex.hui@unsw.edu.au

D. Shu et al. (eds.), *Current Advances in Optometry*, Current Practices in Ophthalmology, https://doi.org/10.1007/978-981-97-8140-9_8

material science behind contact lenses before detailing some of the methods and means through which contact lenses have been investigated to deliver drugs to the eye.

2 Contact Lenses: Overview

2.1 Types of Contact Lenses and Their Classification

Contact lenses have traditionally been classified and considered by practitioners according to their mechanical properties and water content. Durable, rigid corneal lenses (RCLs) (previously more commonly known as rigid gas permeable (RGP) lenses were contrasted primarily with soft contact lenses (SCLs) as the two primary contact lenses prescribed. This has been changing more recently, with other types of lenses outside of these two groups becoming more common, including large, rigid scleral lenses to treat more advanced conditions. While rigid contact lenses are mainly composed of hydrophobic poly methyl methacrylate (PMMA), siloxy methacrylate, cellulose acetate butyrate, or more recently, fluoro-siloxy methacrylates, soft contact lenses are based on flexible hydrophilic polymers such as poly hydroxyethyl methacrylate (pHEMA) and polyvinyl alcohol (PVA). pHEMA-based SCLs are the most popular CLs used in practice due to a combination of water content, oxygen permeability, and comfort of use [4]. Oxygen transmission through contact lenses is also a significant factor to their long-term biocompatibility. The lens thickness has a significant influence on oxygen permeability of SCLs, thus, as the lens thickness approaches 0.1 mm, oxygen transmissibility decreases sharply which can cause hypoxia, particularly during extended wear overnight when the eye is closed. The incorporation of silicone into both RCLs and SCLs has been important for physiological compatibility to try to address this issue, resulting in design of silicone hydrogel soft contact lenses in which poly dimethyl siloxane, tris-trimethylsiloxy silyl, or tris(trimethylsiloxy)-methacryloxy propyl silane are copolymerized with hydroxyethyl methacrylate, *N,N*-dimethylacrylamide, or *N*-vinyl pyrrolidone [4]. Incorporation of silicone allows for the fabrication of contact lenses with higher oxygen permeability, making them suitable for extended wear. Without silicone, oxygen transmissibility in soft contact lenses is solely dependent on the water content. pHEMA, PVA and silicone hydrogel contact lenses currently account for approximately 88% of the contact lens market worldwide, with silicone hydrogel CLs holding the largest share at around 64% [5, 6]. Depending on the composition, SCLs offer a wide range of physical and mechanical properties. For example, while silicone hydrogels are typically very oxygen permeable, and pHEMA shows good oxygen permeability, PVA is of low oxygen permeability. pHEMA and PVA are also hydrophilic, but silicone-based contact lenses are hydrophobic. At the same time, silicone CLs are of high modulus and durable, pHEMA is flexible and PVA is of high tensile strength. Also, pHEMA is prone to protein absorption, but PVA CLs are known to be antibiofouling [7]. pHEMA can also be copolymerized with other highly hydrophilic monomers such as *N*-vinyl

Table 1 Food and Drug Administration classification of the soft contact lenses

Low water content (<50%) High water content (>50%)	Nonionic
Low water content (<50%) High water content (>50%)	Ionic
—	Silicone hydrogel

pyrrolidone and methacrylic acid to modify properties such as surface friction or lens tribology to further customize desired lens parameters [8].

In general, as SCLs are more popular and provide better patient comfort compared to RCLs, they have been the focal point of TCL research [9–11]. The Food and Drug Administration (FDA) classifies SCLs in five groups as identified in Table 1 [12].

The purpose of this classification scheme is to inform the practitioners of protein deposition behavior as well as compatibility with care and cleaning solutions. They also appear to also be useful in explaining some drug delivery behavior when materials encounter different types of pharmaceuticals. For example, incorporation of components such as methacrylic acid leads to overall negative ionic charged lenses and increases the loading of cationic drugs through ion-ligand interactions. Other drugs may interact mainly with the hydrophilic or hydrophobic components in a therapeutic soft contact lens, leading to certain drug-lens combinations being more favorable for drug loading and potential for sustained drug release [8].

2.1.1 Material Criteria and Selection for CLs and TCLs

Selection of the component mixture for SCL fabrication is critical to ensure proper physical and mechanical properties. Optical transparency, glass transition temperature, oxygen permeability, wettability, and water content are among the most influential physical properties which are required to be optimized for successful contact lens application. Mechanical properties such as the friction of the surface, structural hardness or modulus, and mechanical stability, also need to be considered for efficient synthesis on a mass scale as well as to ensure lenses can maintain the curvatures needed to correct refractive error [4, 7]. To this, additional polymers or oligomers may need to be added when considering drug delivery applications and the challenge is for these additions to not compromise the essential properties of the contact lens while also achieving desired pharmaceutical delivery [13]. For example, a contact lens is required to be placed on the ocular surface, so any additions in pursuit of drug delivery purposes must also be biocompatible without exception. When selecting both the primary components and the drug carriers for a therapeutic contact lens, biocompatibility of the materials and their degradation products (in the case of biodegradable materials) is a crucial factor to consider. A drug delivering contact lens continues to need to be comfortable to wear, stable at physiological temperature and optically clear, and all of these must be taken into consideration by researchers in this area as they try to add in pharmaceutical delivery. Selection of the therapeutic molecules also must be done with care. Some biologically active molecules or drugs may not be stable or may lose their desired function when exposed to physiological temperature or pH, or when exposed to light, or if they are required to go through the contact lens synthesis process which may involve higher temperatures or shorter frequencies of light [14].

For instance, ciprofloxacin, an antibiotic, is poorly soluble in water but soluble in other solvents. Unfortunately, utilization of an appropriate ciprofloxacin solvent can cause significant swelling and damage to the contact lens if they are added together. To address this issue, Liu Z. et al. used a water/ethanol solvent system and demonstrated that adding up to 25 vol/vol% of water to ethanol significantly controlled swelling of the lens. Furthermore, this approach improved the loading and release profile of the drug, and demonstrated the type of troubleshooting, which is inherent to adding drug delivery properties to lenses [15]. Challenges related to material selection for therapeutic contact lens design may vary depending on the intrinsic properties of the contact lens, such as solvent vulnerability and hydrophilicity and may preclude specific combinations of lens materials and certain drugs. In addition, other considerations include durability of the components with respect to length of wear and manufacturing cost, which collectively impact commercialization of the therapeutic contact lens [7].

Consideration also must be made on how the TCL will be used. The delivery of different drugs may require appropriate timing and dosing profiles, ranging from continuous, 'zero-order' delivery for short-lived drugs such as pilocarpine, to high initial doses followed by a sustained lower dose for anti-inflammatory drug applications such as corticosteroids [14]. The delivery time course also impacts selection of contact lens materials and replacement frequencies. Daily disposable contact lenses may not be the best option for long-term drug release if they need to be worn continuously. Furthermore, physical properties of the contact lenses used for drug delivery have a significant effect on amount of drug loading based on the power dependent thickness of the lens. For instance, incorporating active monomers into a contact lens may result in excessive cross-linking and thus alter the optical and swelling behavior of the lens [16].

Designing TCLs that are safe, comfortable, and meet demands of a specific application often requires combining properties of two or more components. For example, Maria Vivero-Lopez et al. attempted to combine the antibiofouling property of phosphorylcholine with the antioxidant and prebiotic effects of resveratrol in a CL by copolymerizing 2-hydroxyethyl methacrylate (HEMA) with 2-methacryloyloxyethyl phosphorylcholine (MPCAs). They showed that homogeneous distribution of MPC along the pHEMA hydrogel depth caused a remarkable increase in free water content and decreased Young's modulus. Interestingly, MPC did not show any adverse effect on the uptake of resveratrol by the CLs and had network/water partition coefficients of >100. The resulting pHEMA contact lens showed reduced growth colonies of *P. aeruginosa* and *S. aureus*, anti-inflammatory properties, and biocompatibility as evidenced by in vivo studies in rabbit tests [6].

2.1.2 Drug Loading Strategies for Sustained Release from CLs

Various loading strategies have been developed to incorporate drugs in contact lenses for therapeutic purposes, each with its own advantages and limitations and will be presented in this section. Some research groups have designed specific lens formulations to fabricate TCLs [11, 12], while others have focused on developing drug loading methods for commercially available lens formulations (with slight modifications). The latter approach could potentially be more feasible for commercialization as they use materials which are already available on the market.

2.1.3 Soaking

One of the simplest drug loading methods used in the preparation of therapeutic contact lenses is soaking, which is a cost-effective, and widely used approach, particularly for hydrogel contact lenses. This method involves immersing a pre-formed contact lens in a drug solution, allowing for drug diffusion into the lens via a concentration difference (known as osmotic pressure). Alternatively, eye drop instillation on a contact lens worn by the patient can also be used, although, sustained release from the lens via this method is questionable [17]. When a therapeutic contact lens is worn by a patient, drug release occurs via diffusion through pathways in the contact lens to the tear film, both in the pre and post lens tear space. The overall loading capacity of the contact lens in soaking depends on several factors, such as drug concentration in the loading medium, lens thickness, hydrophilicity of the drug, presence of hydrophilic/hydrophobic components in the lens, molecular weight/size of the drug, lens incubation time, and water content [10]. However, it should be noted that loading drugs can cause alteration of the lens critical properties including increased swelling and decreased optical transparency, and in general, soaking methods suffer from low drug loading and an uncontrolled, large initial burst release of the drug of interest [10]. Chemical and environmental conditions, such as concentration, pH, and temperature, can be adjusted to optimize loading capacity, to some degree [10]. Innovative methods have been developed to address some of the shortcomings of soaking, to try and increase drug loading or extend its release. For example, Pluronic® F-68, a nonionic surfactant, has been used to dissolve gatifloxacin precipitates in the contact lens matrix, leading to improved drug uptake. This approach resulted in acceptable swelling ratios (92.36%) and optical transparency (92.84%) at carefully optimized levels and ratios of gatifloxacin to Pluronic [18]. The presence of the surfactant also supported sustained release of gatifloxacin for up to 72 h from these lenses, as evidenced both by in vitro and in vivo experiments in a rabbit model [18].

2.2 Modified Materials and Soaking Techniques

2.2.1 Pre-loading with Graphene Oxide or Gold Nanoparticles

Pre-loading of nanoparticles into the lens material itself has been found to be an effective strategy for increasing drug loading, reducing burst release, and prolonging the sustained release period [19]. Maulvi et al. used nanotechnology to address the issues associated with loading hydrophobic drugs through soaking.

Bimatoprost: The researchers added bimatoprost and graphene oxide (GO) to a silicone hydrogel contact lens formulation during the polymerization step. This led to a significant increase in the drug loading capacity and a sustained release period of bimatoprost. The GO-containing contact lenses were also transparent, with over 92% transparency, after loading with bimatoprost through soaking. This was attributed to the efficient dispersion of the drug molecules on the GO surface within the lens matrix. Additionally, the water retention power of the GO nanoparticles improved the swelling property of the drug-loaded composite contact lens [19].

Timolol: A similar strategy has been seen using gold nanoparticles. Silicone hydrogel contact lenses were pre-loaded with gold nanoparticles (GNPs) during manufacturing (GNPs-CL) and through soaking (GNPs-SS). The contact lenses were then soaked in timolol solutions of two different concentrations (2 and 4 mg/ml). The addition of the gold nanoparticles did not affect the swelling and optical transmittance of the contact lenses, but the timolol loading significantly increased using GNPs using both approaches. In vitro release profiles of timolol remained almost unchanged for both methods, but in vivo measurements in rabbit tear fluid showed higher timolol concentration with the GNPs-laden contact lenses at all time points compared to those without GNPs. In vivo pharmacodynamic studies showed a remarkable decrease in intraocular pressure (IOP) over 72 h using the GNPs-laden contact lenses, whereas soaked contact lenses without GNPs and eye drop solutions (0.5%w/v) only showed a decrease of 2 mmHg that lasted for only 12 h. Furthermore, the drug deposition in the ciliary body significantly increased with the GNPs-laden contact lenses, suggesting that incorporation of nanoparticles into these lenses may lead to more of the timolol being bioavailable at the desired sites of action [20].

2.2.2 Incorporation of Vitamin E

Pre-loading of Vitamin E on to the surface of lenses is another potential strategy to address the short release time associated with soaking. By pre-loading hydrogel contact lenses with Vitamin E, a hydrophobic molecule with antioxidant properties, the release duration of both hydrophobic and hydrophilic drugs can be increased through different mechanisms. The drug can dissolve into the Vitamin E to form a "drug depot" or diffuse through an increased pathway created by the Vitamin E barrier. It has also been reported that Vitamin E pre-loading enhances the stability of the loaded drugs. Both drug loading and release time (ranging from a few hours to a few days) can be adjusted as a function of Vitamin E loading and the solvent system used for pre-loading, while transparency of the loaded contact lenses remains only minimally affected for a range of ophthalmic agents, including timolol, cyclosporine, and dexamethasone [15].

2.2.3 Host–Guest Inclusion Complexes

The generation of host–guest inclusion complexes, where specific molecules such as cyclodextrins are used to interact with drugs of interest, increasing both their loading and solubility, has also been utilized to enhance the efficiency of soaking in ocular drug delivery. These can be particularly useful in allowing for meaningful loading of drugs which have poor aqueous solubility such as many of the antifungal agents. For instance, econazole/hydroxypropyl-alpha-cyclodextrin and econazole/hydroxypropyl-beta-cyclodextrin inclusion complexes were prepared and loaded into soft hydrogel contact lenses through soaking, and then applied to freshly enucleated porcine eyeballs. The hydrogel contact lenses and the hydrogel contact lenses loaded with the cyclodextrin inclusion complexes delivered 2.8 and 5 times more drug across the corneas, respectively, compared to econazole nitrate eye drops at the same concentrations. Furthermore, while the eye drop led to concentrations below the minimum inhibitory concentration (MIC) of the drug against test agents of *Fusarium semitectum* and *Fusarium solani* (141 μg/mL) and *Scolecobasidium tshawytschae* and *Bipolaris hawaiiensis* (283 μg/mL), the hydrogels containing the inclusion complexes demonstrated efficient antifungal activity against these fungi, suggesting a potential application in the treatment of keratitis [21].

2.2.4 Molecular Imprinting

Molecular imprinting enables chemical or physical interactions between specific sites on the hydrogel and the drug through generation of molecular memory within the final polymer. This is achieved through incorporation of molecules in the synthesis process which are similar to the target drug of interest, creating both size and functional group specific areas within the materials and have been used for a variety of studies with contact lenses [10]. High degrees of cross-linking are necessary for this technique to be successful, as there is some degree of mechanical strength required for the final polymer to be able to efficiently and effectively interact with the drug of interest [10]. Molecular imprinting techniques have begun to consider the known chemical structures of drugs or receptors in the selection of components to be included in the mixtures. Inspired by the activity of statins as 3-hydroxy-3-methylglutaryl–CoA (HMG–CoA) reductase inhibitors, Pereira-da-Mota et al. designed pHEMA hydrogel lenses using ethylene glycol phenyl ether methacrylate (EGPEM), 2-aminoethyl methacrylate hydrochloride (AEMA), and *N*-(3-aminopropyl) methacrylamide hydrochloride (APMA) as the comonomers with functional groups to resemble those of HMG–CoA. Copolymerization with AEMA and APMA increased the loading capacity of the contact lenses for atorvastatin, and atorvastatin accumulation in these materials reached levels sufficient for the treatment of ocular surface diseases, as evidenced by permeability studies using porcine cornea and sclera tissues [22]. Similarly, González-Chomón C. et al. developed a contact lens with an affinity to olopatadine, an antihistaminic drug, by mimicking the composition of the natural H1-receptor to which olopatadine behaves as an antagonist. They used acrylic acid, 2-acrylamido-2-methyl-1-propanesulfonic acid, and benzyl methacrylate as comonomers to fabricate a hydrogel CL with a high capacity for olopatadine. The drug-loaded CL passed both the biocompatibility test with mast cells and the HET-CAM test of ocular irritancy successfully [23] It should be noted however, the high degree of cross-linking in molecular imprinting can sometimes alter the optical and physical characteristics of the contact lenses [16].

2.2.5 Supercritical Fluid Impregnation and Deposition

The supercritical fluid impregnation (SFI) method utilizes a supercritical solvent, such as carbon dioxide, to carry the drug into a pre-formed polymeric matrix such as a contact lens. The supercritical solvent plasticizes the polymeric matrix and causes it to swell, which allows for the mobile phase containing the drug to diffuse more quickly. When pressure is released, the drug is deposited into the polymer via two main mechanisms: by dispersing molecularly in the contact lens material (SFI) or by precipitating within the hydrogel (supercritical fluid deposition or SFD). Addition of small amounts of cosolvents can enhance the process by increasing solvent polarity, promoting drug solubility, or by increasing polymer swelling and pliability. Therefore, the amount of impregnated or dispersed drug can be regulated by altering process conditions such as pressure and temperature, selecting suitable cosolvents, and varying their compositions. While SFI results in a release profile similar to that of soaking, SFD enables elongated and sustained release of the drug [8].

A recent study showed that it is possible to create therapeutic contact lenses with acetazolamide and timolol maleate using solvent mixtures of supercritical carbon dioxide with ethanol or water ($scCO_2$ + EtOH and $scCO_2$ + H_2O). The amount of impregnated drug can vary depending on the type and concentration of cosolvent used (in addition to operational conditions such as temperature and pressure), which can be useful for controlling drug amounts for drugs with different hydrophilic/hydrophobic character [24]. This technology has shown promise in improving drug loading capacity and release duration for both hydrophilic and hydrophobic drugs. However, the process can be expensive and time-consuming [25].

2.2.6 Drug-Loaded Nanocarriers

Nanoparticles have a large surface area-to-volume ratio, which enables them to efficiently encapsulate drugs and release them over an extended period. In contact lenses, drug-loaded nanoparticles can be incorporated into the lens material or coated onto the surface, leading to prolonged release. The size and drug loading of the nanoparticles are crucial factors in determining the drug release rate and duration. Additionally, various types of nanoparticles, such as polymeric, colloidal, or lipid-based, can be utilized to optimize drug delivery in contact lenses. Figure 1 illustrates the structures of nanoparticles commonly utilized in therapeutic contact lenses. Additionally, the nanocarriers themselves can play a protective role against biological conditions, potentially leading to increased drug stability under various conditions encountered in storage or on the ocular surface. This property, along with high bioavailability and extended residence time make nanocarriers attractive candidates for drug-eluting contact lenses. Different nanoparticle carriers have been prepared and evaluated as delivery systems for a broad range of eye complications using a variety of agents. Table 2 summarizes the most common nanoparticle systems in TCLs, along with a schematic display of structural features of each group.

2.2.7 Cyclodextrin Inclusion Sites

Cyclodextrins (CDs) are cyclic oligosaccharides widely used in the pharmaceutical industry. Biologically safe CDs consist of 6–8 glucose units that form a hydrophobic interior cavity with a hydrophilic exterior, known as α-CD (6 glucose units), β-CD (7 glucose units), and γ-CD (8 glucose units). CDs are excellent candidates

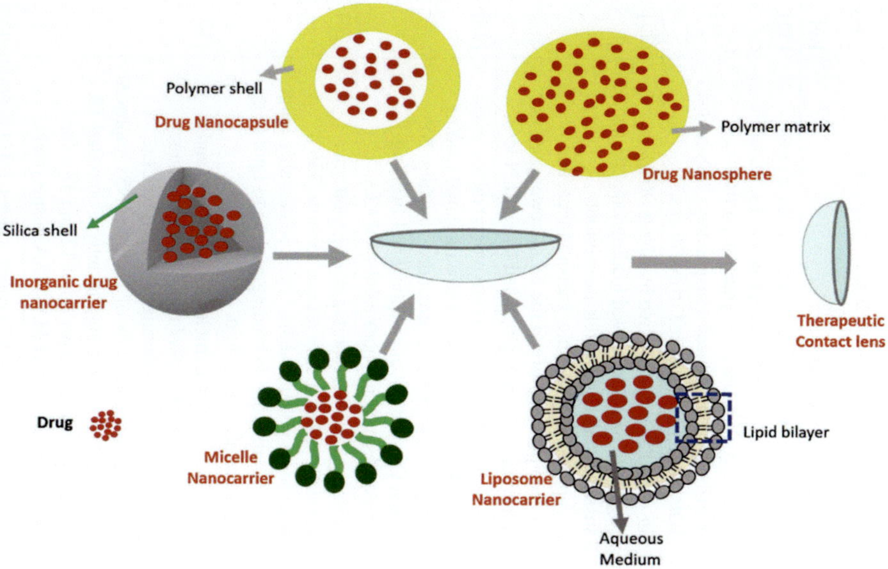

Fig. 1 Drug-loaded nanostructures incorporated into therapeutic contact lenses

for drug reservoirs/carriers due to their structural specifications. Hydrophobic and water-insoluble drugs can form complexes with CDs to create release systems of high loading capacity that support an extended-release period into hydrophilic environments such as the ocular surface (Fig. 2a) [31]. For drug delivery and tissue regeneration purposes, CDs can be chemically conjugated to the contact lens material, applied as a coating through self-assembly, or simply mixed with drug-loaded CDs.

Recently, an antibacterial coating was applied to the surface of a CL through layer-by-layer (LBL) electrostatic self-assembly was combined with host–guest inclusion to treat bacterial keratitis. The LBL self-assembly method is commonly used for surface modification and creating multilayer films with precise control over thickness, making it an eco-friendly manufacturing process. It can be used to modify almost any substrate surface, including CLs, and has been used to create sustained release CLs.

To combine these two techniques, the polyanionic copolymer P(AA-*co*-AdA) (PAcA) was synthesized by radical copolymerization of acrylic acid (AA) and 1-adamantan-1-ylmethyl acrylate (AdA) and combined with poly(ethyleneimine) (PEI) to enable layer-by-layer (LBL) self-assembly on the surface of the CLs. Next, β-cyclodextrin-levofloxacin (β-CD-LEV) was used to prepare an antibacterial coating through AdA/β-CD-LEV host–guest interaction. The antibacterial and germicidal efficacy were shown in vitro and in vivo in an animal model of staphylococcal keratitis. Also, the coated contact lens showed optical transparency, in vitro. The drug loading capacity and thickness of the coating layer can be controlled through the host–guest recognition time and number of the layers. The authors believe that

Table 2 Examples of nanoparticle systems used as drug carrier in TCLs

Nanoparticle	NP preparation method	Lens material	Drug(s)	Disease	Results and significance	Ref.
mPEG-PLA Micelle	Thin film hydration	pHEMA; free radical polymerization of HEMA+NPs	Timolol and latanoprost	Glaucoma	In vivo (in rabbits) release was sustained for timolol (120 h) and latanoprost (96 h); micelles exhibited ultra-small size/narrow particle size distribution and optical transparency; 9.8× higher IOP reduction compared to eye drops.	[26]
PEGylated SLN	Solvent evaporation	pHEMA(+DMA); free radical polymerization; soaked in NPs suspension in STF, for 10 days	Latanoprost	Glaucoma	In vitro 120 h, and in vivo in rabbits 96 h; pegylated SLNs improved loading capacity and sustained latanoprost release without compromising swelling, transmittance, and oxygen permeability of the CLs. Lower protein adherence than non-pegylated laden SLN lens.	[27]
Silica shell nanoparticle-laden	Microemulsion	pHEMA(+MAA); free radical polymerization; monomers+ NPs	Ketotifen	Ocular Allergy	240 h in vitro, and 240 h in vivo in rabbits' eyes; extended drug delivery even with initial loading (65 μg). In contrast to direct drug loading, NPs laden CLs did not alter optical and swelling properties, and ion permeability of CLs.	[28]
Drug-loaded Eudragit S100 NPs laden	Quasi-emulsion solvent diffusion technique	pHEMA(+MAA, NVP); CLs consisted drug laden ring and drug free center	Cyclosporine	Chronic dry eye syndrome	No drug loss was reported during monomer extraction, 168 h drug release in vitro, 336 h release, in vivo in rabbits' eyes, remarkably longer than in vitro, due to binding of drug to lipid (e.g., cholesterol) in tear fluid.	[29]
Poloxamer40/ PVA stabilized nano-suspensions (NSs)	Controlled precipitation	Two CLs: 1. pHEMA (+MAA) radical solution polymerization, 2. Hilafilcon B (pHEMA (+NVP)	Triamcinolone acetonide	Ocular inflammation	NSs with a mean particle size of 147 nm and a drug load of 0.8 mg/ml using PVA/poloxamer stabilizer, had no blurring effect on the CLs. Increased concentration of TA in the NSs improved the drug-loaded dose significantly. Controlled TA release profiles for a period of 12 and 48 h for Hilafilcon B and pHEMA-MAA, respectively.	[30]

PEG poly(ethylene glycol), *pHEMA* poly(2-hydroxyethyl methacrylate), *IOP* intraocular pressure, *SLN* solid lipid NPs, *NPs* nanoparticles, *DMA N,N*-dimethyl acrylamide, *MAA* methacrylic acid, *NVP N*-vinylpyrrolidone, *NSs* nanospheres, *TA* Triamcinolone acetonide, *PVA* poly(vinyl alcohol)

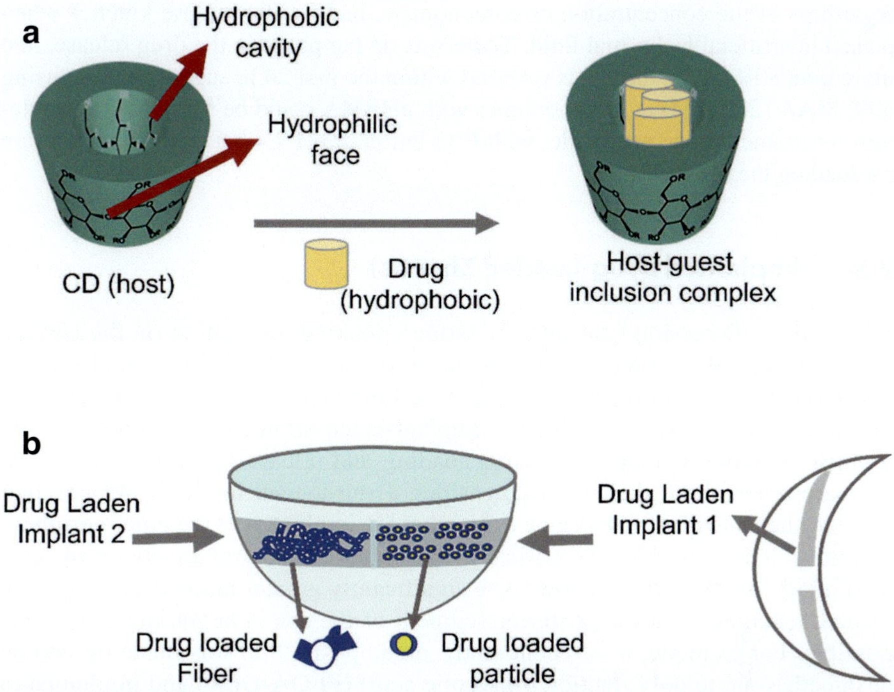

Fig. 2 (**a**) Host–guest inclusion complex formation between CDs ad hydrophobic drugs; (**b**) Contact lens with drug-loaded implants

the adhered dead bacteria can be release and reloading of β-CD-LEV can be achieved through immersion in a LEV solution [32].

2.2.8 Drug Loading Based on Electrostatic Interactions

Electrostatic interactions have also been tapped to improve drug loading and extend delivery, so long as there are appropriate charged species of the drug of interest to interact with an oppositely charged lens material. García-Millán et al. conducted a study on how modifying the chemical and structural properties of pHEMA contact lenses affect the loading and release of triamcinolone acetonide, a corticosteroid drug. They investigated two types of lenses, one made with NVP as a comonomer and the other with MAA as a comonomer. They used saline solution and PBS buffer solution (pH of 7.4) for drug loading and found that the lenses had similar swelling properties in saline solution, but in PBS buffer, the contact lens with MAA as a comonomer had enhanced swelling compared to the one with NVP. This was due to the carboxylic groups in MAA, which become ionized at pH 7.4, causing the hydrogel to swell. The use of comonomers increased the amount of drug loaded in the lens, and the swelling properties affected the drug loading in PBS buffer. The lens with 40% MAA (200 mM) showed the most efficient drug loading when PBS buffer was used as the loading solution. The release profiles showed that all the lenses, regardless of the concentration of comonomers, had similar release kinetics when placed in artificial lachrymal fluid. There was no lag phase in the drug release, and more than 80% of the drug was released within the first 24 h, suggesting that using 40% MAA (200 mM) as a comonomer with pHEMA could be a potential formulation for triamcinolone acetonide, with PBS buffer at pH 7.4 being an ideal medium for loading the drug [33].

2.3 Implanted Drug-Loaded Sheet(s)

Simple drug dispersion (during fabrication), soaking, or coating on the surface has the potential to compromise critical properties such as mechanical properties, oxygen or ion permeability and may be limited in drug loading capacity and ultimate drug release. Drug-loaded implant-laden strategies, in contrast, hold promise to address some of the drug loading and release limitations, however, they are not without their own downsides. Drug-loaded implants are polymer films or sheets loaded with drug carriers that are implanted in the outer periphery of contact lenses, leaving the critical properties of the central area (over the cornea) intact. As these films allow for a significantly greater amount of drug to be loaded, reaching even the posterior segment of the eye is beginning to become possible. For example, in a recent study, a composite film was made by adding dexamethasone to poly (lactic-*co*-glycolic acid) (PLGA-DEX) and implanted in the outer periphery of a pHEMA methafilcon-based soft contact lens. By incorporating a large amount of dexamethasone into this composite film, in vivo application of these lenses on rabbits led to a 200-fold increase in drug concentration at the retina compared to the intensive hourly eye drop instillation, all while having significantly lower with a lower drug concentration in the blood serum suggesting a superior systemic safety profile. Additionally, an efficacy study in rabbits revealed the inhibitory effect of the worn contact lenses on retinal vascular leakage induced by intravitreal injection of vascular endothelial growth factor (VEGF). A 4-week follow-up confirmed the safety of the drug-eluting contact lenses in healthy rabbits [34].

Drug-loaded sheets also have the capacity for multiple drug delivery (Fig. 2b). In some patients with glaucoma, single drug therapy may not effectively control intraocular pressure (IOP), and some combination of IOP lowering eye drops is often prescribed. A multiple implant-laden silicone hydrogel contact lens (IM) has been developed to passively deliver timolol, bimatoprost, and hyaluronic acid. During dry radiation sterilization and hydration for 24 h prior to use, the drugs showed a loss 16.87%, 47.95%, and 24.41% for timolol, bimatoprost, and HA, respectively. In vitro experiments showed a significantly lower burst of drug release as well as an elongated sustained release of the drugs (up to 72 h) compared to soaked and direct drug-included contact lenses, with the authors suggesting that the decrease in burst could reduce the risk of side effects. The implanted contact lenses led to a prolonged reduction in IOP for 120 h, in contrast to the peak and valley profile seen with multiple eye drop instillations [35].

3 Current Commercialization and Future Application of Therapeutic Contact Lenses in the Management of Ocular Diseases

The arguments for the development and research into drug-eluting contact lenses center on the ubiquity of CLs having been safely worn by millions of users worldwide over the last decades and the presumed pharmacokinetic advantages of such a system compared to eye drops. In addition, therapeutic contact lenses can function as a reservoir of preservative free drug that can remain in contact with the cornea and thus facilitate ocular treatment of the drug so long as it is worn. The first drug releasing contact lens has reached the market, specifically targeting the management of ocular allergy with a daily disposable ketotifen releasing contact lens [23]. A vast group of commercial silicone hydrogels, conventional hydrogels, and daily disposable contact lenses have been demonstrated to support sustained release of ketotifen fumarate at a clinically relevant amount compared to conventional eye drops when tested in vitro [36]. Ultimately, etafilcon A, which is a HEMA-based soft contact lens, was utilized by Johnson & Johnson Vision Care to produce a daily-wear, disposable, vision-correcting soft contact lens loaded with 0.019 mg ketotifen and released to the market as Acuvue Theravision. This formulation became the first drug-eluting contact lens to pass different phases of clinical trials successfully and received FDA approval for the prevention of ocular itch due to allergic conjunctivitis [37, 38]. Glaucoma releasing contact lenses are also in clinical trials. LLT-BMT1, a contact lens printed with bimatoprost, has shown promising results in a Phase IIb clinical study conducted by MediPrint™ Ophthalmics' SIGHT-1 clinical program. The product was well-tolerated by patients, and there was a lower incidence of hyperemia compared to bimatoprost drops. The company has initiated [5] a Phase IIb study for dosage optimization called SIGHT-2 and hopes to obtain dose results by the first half of 2023, which will take the clinical study to the Phase III trial. As further contact lens drug delivery devices become commercialized, acceptance of these forms of alternative methods of treatment will become more of a reality for prescribing practitioners and patients and will hopefully lead to improved patient outcomes in treating these diseases [39, 40].

4 Conclusion

The potential for soft contact lenses, due to their water content in comparison with rigid contact lenses, to deliver drugs was identified in the original patents for the materials in the 1960s [41]. Research has continued in this area to demonstrate the potential of these drug delivery devices within the laboratory with a variety of drugs, materials, and testing conditions as well as work in vivo in animals or humans. Matching of a material, drug, drug release kinetics, and disease to be treated will be crucial things to identify for the future success of these devices, and the hope is that the work published in the field will allow for this to be a successful means of ocular drug delivery.

References

1. Mofidfar M, Abdi B, Ahadian S, Mostafavi E, Desai TA, Abbasi F, et al. Drug delivery to the anterior segment of the eye: a review of current and future treatment strategies. Int J Pharm. 2021;607:120924.
2. Baudouin C. Detrimental effect of preservatives in eyedrops: implications for the treatment of glaucoma. Acta Ophthalmol. 2008;86(7):716–26.
3. Farkouh A, Frigo P, Czejka M. Systemic side effects of eye drops: a pharmacokinetic perspective. Clin Ophthalmol. 2016;10:2433–41.
4. Musgrave CSA, Fang F. Contact lens materials: a materials science perspective. Materials (Basel). 2019;12(2):261.
5. Akbari E, Imani R, Shokrollahi P, Heidari KS. Preparation of nanoparticle-containing ring-implanted poly(vinyl alcohol) contact lens for sustained release of hyaluronic acid. Macromol Biosci. 2021;21(7):e2100043.
6. Vivero-Lopez M, Pereira-da-Mota AF, Carracedo G, Huete-Toral F, Parga A, Otero A, et al. Phosphorylcholine-based contact lenses for sustained release of resveratrol: design, antioxidant and antimicrobial performances, and in vivo behavior. Acs Appl Mater Interfaces. 2022;14(50):55431–46.
7. Zhu Y, Li S, Li J, Falcone N, Cui Q, Shah S, et al. Lab-on-a-contact lens: recent advances and future opportunities in diagnostics and therapeutics. Adv Mater. 2022;34(24):e2108389.
8. Xu J, Xue Y, Hu G, Lin T, Gou J, Yin T, et al. A comprehensive review on contact lens for ophthalmic drug delivery. J Control Release. 2018;281:97–118.
9. Bhamra TS, Tighe BJ. Mechanical properties of contact lenses: the contribution of measurement techniques and clinical feedback to 50 years of materials development. Cont Lens Anterior Eye. 2017;40(2):70–81.
10. Rykowska I, Nowak I, Nowak R. Soft contact lenses as drug delivery systems: a review. Molecules. 2021;26(18):5577.
11. Choi SW, Kim J. Therapeutic contact lenses with polymeric vehicles for ocular drug delivery: a review. Materials. 2018;11(7):1125.
12. Peral A, Martinez-Aguila A, Pastrana C, Huete-Toral F, Carpena-Torres C, Carracedo G. Contact lenses as drug delivery system for glaucoma: a review. Appl Sci. 2020;10(15):5151.
13. Jones L, Hui A, Phan CM, Read ML, Azar D, Buch J, et al. CLEAR-contact lens technologies of the future. Cont Lens Anterior Eye. 2021;44(2):398–430.
14. Novack GD, Barnett M. Ocular drug delivery systems using contact lenses. J Ocul Pharmacol Ther. 2020;36(8):595–601.
15. Liu Z, Overton M, Chauhan A. Transport of vitamin E from ethanol/water solution into contact lenses and impact on drug transport. J Ocul Pharmacol Ther. 2022;38(6):396–403.
16. Maulvi FA, Singhania SS, Desai AR, Shukla MR, Tannk AS, Ranch KM, et al. Contact lenses with dual drug delivery for the treatment of bacterial conjunctivitis. Int J Pharm. 2018;548(1):139–50.
17. Alvarez-Lorenzo C, Anguiano-Igea S, Varela-Garcia A, Vivero-Lopez M, Concheiro A. Bioinspired hydrogels for drug-eluting contact lenses. Acta Biomater. 2019;84:49–62.
18. Maulvi FA, Parmar RJ, Desai AR, Desai DM, Shukla MR, Ranch KM, et al. Tailored gatifloxacin Pluronic(R) F-68-loaded contact lens: addressing the issue of transmittance and swelling. Int J Pharm. 2020;581:119279.
19. Maulvi FA, Soni PD, Patel PJ, Desai AR, Desai DT, Shukla MR, et al. Controlled bimatoprost release from graphene oxide laden contact lenses: in vitro and in vivo studies. Colloids Surf B: Biointerfaces. 2021;208:112096.
20. Maulvi FA, Patil RJ, Desai AR, Shukla MR, Vaidya RJ, Ranch KM, et al. Effect of gold nanoparticles on timolol uptake and its release kinetics from contact lenses: in vitro and in vivo evaluation. Acta Biomater. 2019;86:350–62.

21. Wong A, Fallon M, Celiksoy V, Ferla S, Varricchio C, Whitaker D, et al. A composite system based upon hydroxypropyl cyclodextrins and soft hydrogel contact lenses for the delivery of therapeutic doses of econazole to the cornea, in vitro. Pharmaceutics. 2022;14(8):1631.
22. Pereira-da-Mota AF, Vivero-Lopez M, Topete A, Serro AP, Concheiro A, Alvarez-Lorenzo C. Atorvastatin-eluting contact lenses: effects of molecular imprinting and sterilization on drug loading and release. Pharmaceutics. 2021;13(5):606.
23. González-Chomón C, Silva M, Concheiro A, Alvarez-Lorenzo C. Biomimetic contact lenses eluting olopatadine for allergic conjunctivitis. Acta Biomater. 2016;41:302–11.
24. Costa VP, Braga ME, Duarte CM, Alvarez-Lorenzo C, Concheiro A, Gil MH, et al. Anti-glaucoma drug-loaded contact lenses prepared using supercritical solvent impregnation. J Supercrit Fluids. 2010;53(1–3):165–73.
25. Xu J, Xue Y, Hu G. A comprehensive review on contact lens for ophthalmic drug delivery. J Control Release. 2018;10(281):97–118.
26. Xu JW, Ge Y, Bu RX, Zhang AN, Feng SS, Wang J, et al. Co-delivery of latanoprost and timolol from micelles-laden contact lenses for the treatment of glaucoma. J Control Release. 2019;305:18–28.
27. Dang H, Dong C, Zhang L. Sustained latanoprost release from PEGylated solid lipid nanoparticle-laden soft contact lens to treat glaucoma. Pharm Dev Technol. 2022;27(2):127–33.
28. Maulvi FA, Mangukiya MA, Patel PA, Vaidya RJ, Koli AR, Ranch KM, et al. Extended release of ketotifen from silica shell nanoparticle-laden hydrogel contact lenses: in vitro and in vivo evaluation. J Mater Sci Mater Med. 2016;27(6):113.
29. Maulvi FA, Choksi HH, Desai AR, Patel AS, Ranch KM, Vyas BA, et al. pH triggered controlled drug delivery from contact lenses: addressing the challenges of drug leaching during sterilization and storage. Colloids Surf B Biointerfaces. 2017;157:72–82.
30. Garcia-Millan E, Quintans-Carballo M, Otero-Espinar FJ. Improved release of triamcinolone acetonide from medicated soft contact lenses loaded with drug nanosuspensions. Int J Pharm. 2017;525(1):226–36.
31. Sun ZX, Zheng L, Wang K, Huai Z, Liu ZR. Primary vs secondary: directionalized guest coordination in beta-cyclodextrin derivatives. Carbohydr Polym. 2022;297:120050.
32. Wen SM, Qin C, Shen LL, Liu D, Zhu SQ, Lin QK. Surface self-assembly construction of therapeutic contact lens with bacterial "kill-releasing" and drug-reloading capabilities for efficient bacterial keratitis treatment. ACS Biomater Sci Eng. 2022;8(3):1329–41.
33. Chatterjee S, Upadhyay P, Mishra M, Srividya M, Akshara MR, Kamali N, et al. Advances in chemistry and composition of soft materials for drug releasing contact lenses. RSC Adv. 2020;10(60):36751–77.
34. Ross AE, Bengani LC, Tulsan R, Maidana DE, Salvador-Culla B, Kobashi H, et al. Topical sustained drug delivery to the retina with a drug-eluting contact lens. Biomaterials. 2019;217:119285.
35. Desai AR, Maulvi FA, Desai DM, et al. Multiple drug delivery from the drug-implants-laden silicone contact lens: Addressing the issue of burst drug release. Mater Sci Eng. 2020;112C:110885.
36. Soluri A, Hui A, Jones L. Delivery of ketotifen fumarate by commercial contact lens materials. Optom Vis Sci. 2012;89(8):1140–9.
37. Ono J, Toshida H. Use of ketotifen fumarate-eluting daily disposable soft contact lens in management of ocular allergy: literature review and report of two cases. Cureus. 2022;14(7):e27093.
38. A drug-eluting contact lens for allergic conjunctivitis. Med Lett Drugs Ther. 2022;64(1648):60–1.
39. Balfour H. Drug-eluting contact lens shows potential in first-in-human study. Eur Pharm Rev. 2021;
40. Ganatra S. MediPrint™ ophthalmics announces it has initiated its SIGHT-2 phase 2b clinical study for its lead asset; 2022.
41. Sedlácek J. Possibility of the application of ophthalmic drugs with the use of gel contact lenses. Cesk Oftalmol. 1965;21(6):509–12.

Novel Ocular Drug Delivery Methods

Yuan Fang, Chris Hodge, Gerard Sutton, and Jingjing You

1 Introduction

There are many challenges involved in ocular drug delivery because of the unique anatomical and physiological factors in the eye. Currently, 90% of all ophthalmic drug formulations are applied as eye drops [1]. However, because of the static barriers (including the cornea, conjunctiva, and sclera) and dynamic barriers (including blinking reflex, high tear turnover rate, and rapid restoration of eye film), less than 5% of the applied dose can penetrate and reach intraocular tissue, leading to low

Y. Fang
School of Medical Sciences, University of Sydney, Camperdown, NSW, Australia
e-mail: yfan8920@uni.sydney.edu.au

C. Hodge
Vision Eye Institute Chatswood, Sydney, NSW, Australia

Save Sight Institute, The University of Sydney, Sydney, NSW, Australia

Graduate School of Health, University of Technology Sydney, Sydney, NSW, Australia

NSW Tissue Bank, Sydney, NSW, Australia
e-mail: christopher.hodge@uts.edu.au

G. Sutton
Vision Eye Institute Chatswood, Sydney, NSW, Australia

Save Sight Institute, The University of Sydney, Sydney, NSW, Australia

NSW Tissue Bank, Sydney, NSW, Australia
e-mail: gerard.sutton@sydney.edu.au

J. You (✉)
School of Medical Sciences, University of Sydney, Camperdown, NSW, Australia

Save Sight Institute, The University of Sydney, Sydney, NSW, Australia
e-mail: jing.you@sydney.edu.au

D. Shu et al. (eds.), *Current Advances in Optometry*, Current Practices in Ophthalmology, https://doi.org/10.1007/978-981-97-8140-9_9

bioavailability of approximately 1–3% [1, 2]. In the initial stages of the application of eye drops, the majority will be washed away by tear production and blinking of the eyes. The remaining drugs will be delivered through the corneal route and non-corneal route as described below (Fig. 1).

The innate structure of the cornea negatively impacts drug penetration. Anatomically, the cornea consists of five layers, from anterior to posterior; corneal epithelium, Bowman's layer, corneal stroma, Descemet's membrane, and corneal endothelium. Each layer has different priorities and potential rate-limiting structures for drug permeability. Among the five structures of the cornea, epithelium and stroma are considered two major drug diffusion barriers. The lipoidal epithelium cells number account for 90% of the total cornea cells, causing a significant resistance to hydrophilic drug permeability. Furthermore, the junctional complex network of epithelium also acts as a barrier to the diffusion of drugs [1]. Corneal stroma constitutes 90% thickness of the cornea that contains aligned cells guided by parallel hydrated collagen lamellae [1]. The hydrophilic nature of stroma makes it a significant barrier for hydrophobic drugs. Although relatively uncommon in practice, if the drugs are targeting the posterior part of the eye, the drug will need to penetrate the cornea, move into the anterior chamber and then through the iris, to the posterior chamber and into posterior tissue. Among these structures, it is mainly the iris-ciliary body and the aqueous humor that prevent further penetration of the drug from corneal

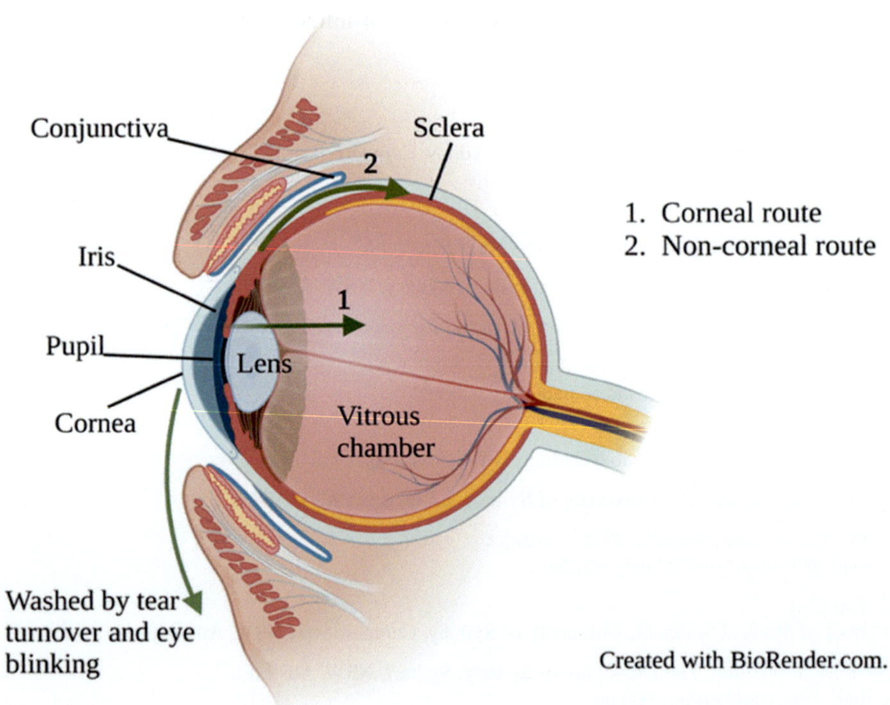

Fig. 1 The routes and barriers in topical administration

absorption. When the drug is distributed in the vascularized iris and ciliary body, it can permeate into the blood vessels and move into the systemic circulation [3]. Drugs in the anterior chamber may also be eliminated through aqueous humor outflow [3].

Understandably therefore, achieving therapeutic concentration levels in the posterior segment is challenging through this long route. The non-cornea drug delivery pathway involves the conjunctiva and sclera. Human conjunctiva is a highly vascular structure with approximately 17 times the surface area of the cornea, which allows macromolecules (with a molecular weight ranging from 1000 to 20,000 Da) to pass through with a permeability coefficient negatively related to solute size [4]. However, a large portion of the drug is absorbed by conjunctival blood capillaries and lymphatics, and entry into system circulation before penetration into the ocular tissue [1]. The sclera is made of connective tissue containing collagen fibers to protect and support the eye, which has comparable drug permeability with corneal stroma and is more permeable for molecules with a smaller radius [1].

The low drug bioavailability of eye drops delivery mandates frequent administration. The highly frequent dosing schedule results in poor patient compliance and may cause side effects in a long term. Although an extreme example, corneal microbial keratitis patients need to instill eye drops every 30 min in the first 24–36 h in mild to moderate cases [5]. Routinely, topical medication for reducing intraoperative pressure may demand instillation between 2 and 4 times per day. The frequent dosing schedule results in poor patient compliance and result in an extended treatment period. Frequent instillation can lead to ocular surface disruption and irritation or stinging on further application. Practically, frequent instillation has been known also cause joint and muscle pain in the application finger, albeit in patients with pre-existing conditions such as arthritis which may limit movement.

Many novel drug delivery systems have been explored to overcome the limitations related to the topical ophthalmic formulation. The ideal drug delivery system requires easy administration, long residence time, high biocompatibility, and does not interfere with vision and normal eye function [2]. In this context, novel hydrogel and nanoparticle drug delivery techniques will be discussed, as they are the most frequently analyzed ocular drug delivery platforms that can be applied for both anterior and posterior segment eye diseases.

2 Hydrogel

To overcome the low bioavailability of topical administration and prevent quickly being washed away from the ocular surface, the hydrogel drug delivery method has been researched. By definition, the hydrogel is a three-dimensional crosslinked polymer network that contains at least 10% water content. Hydrogel can be fabricated from natural polymers such as alginate, collagen, and chitosan, or synthetic polymers such as poly(vinyl alcohol) and poly(hydroxyl alkyl methacrylate) [6].

Natural polymers have the advantages of high biocompatibility and non-toxicity subunits, while potentially limited by their weak mechanical properties [7]. The synthetic polymers are beneficial in the higher batch-to-batch reproductivity and stability, but they are limited by inflammation response and cytotoxic by-products after degradation. Hydrophilic polymers can be chemically or physically crosslinked from liquid to gel to allow a longer residence time and show a sustained drug-releasing profile representing a further possible advantage. Chemical crosslinked gels are formed by covalently crosslinking chemical agents including *N*-hydroxysuccinimide (NHS) and *N*,*N*-(3-dimethylaminopropyl)-*N*-ethylcarbodiimide hydrochloride (EDC), which results in a stable structure [7]. Drug release in the covalent linkage is usually achieved by enzyme degradation. However, the chemical crosslinker is usually cytotoxic and has potential biosafety concerns. Physically crosslinked hydrogel is normally formed by forces including van der Waals, hydrogen bonding, and electronic bonding. Hydrogels formed by physical interactions are typically less stable and are known to be thermally reversible [7].

High initial drug release, also known as burst release of drug molecules, has been a challenge in hydrogel drug delivery (Fig. 2). The typical hydrogel biomaterial has a mesh size range from 5 to 100 nm, which is larger than most small drug molecules (molecular dimensions of 0.5–1.5 nm) [8]. Therefore, after being transferred to the hydrogel drug delivery system in an aqueous environment, small drug molecules can quickly diffuse from the hydrogel network in the swelling process, resulting in an initial burst release. Burst release can result from other reasons such as the desorption of the drug attaching to the surface of hydrogel and the poor distribution of the drug in the network [9]. Silicone hydrogel and Poly(hydroxyethyl methacrylate) (pHEMA) hydrogel show burst release profiles for most ophthalmic drugs with release lasting for a few hours [10]. The burst release phenomenon usually has negative effects, including cause cytotoxicity and tissue irritation in the human body [11]. Therefore, a constant rate of drug release, also referred to as zero-order sustained drug release, is usually the preferred method of drug delivery [9]. For example, the Retisert implant is a zero-order drug delivery system made from silicone polymer and has been approved by Food and Drug Administration (FDA). It is used to treat chronic non-infectious uveitis in the posterior segment of the eye, providing a continuous release of fluocinolone acetonide for about 30 months after surgical implantation at the back of the eye.

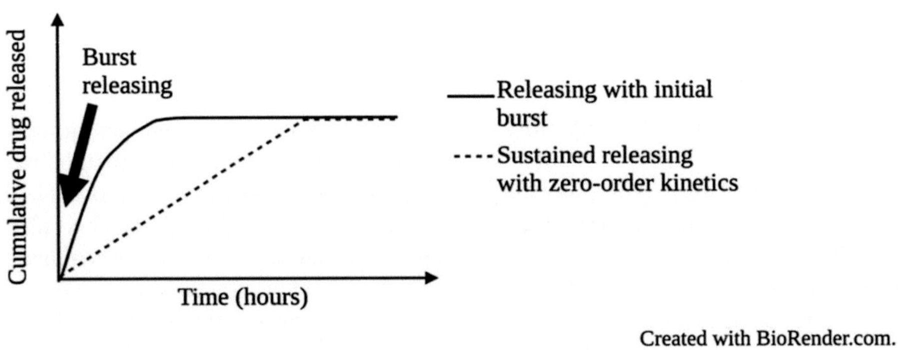

Fig. 2 The illustration of drug release with initial burst and zero-order kinetics

To enhance drug absorption and accomplish sustained and regulated drug release in the hydrogel, it may be necessary to enhance molecule interactions and binding mechanisms within the delivery system. There are various chemical, physical, and biological factors that have been researched to improve drug delivery. Covalent conjugation between the hydrogel polymer and drug can allow a stable binding, which is cleavable through enzyme degradation to allow drug release [6]. The mucoadhesive effect induced by the physical interaction between polymer and mucin can also improve drug delivery. As an example, the mucoadhesive property of chitosan polymer makes it one of the most widely used drug delivery materials [12]. Applying a chitosan-based drug delivery system to the mucosal surface results in an interaction between chitosan and mucin, creating a strong and long-lasting adhesion that facilitates sustained drug release at the site. The physical factors including swelling characteristics and mechanical deformation of the hydrogel can also impact the drug delivery of hydrogel. For instance, encapsulating cyclodextrin in pHEMA hydrogel can lead to an increase in swelling behaviors, resulting in improved drug uptake [13]. With the ability of mechanical deformation from liquid to solid in response to environmental changes, the in situ hydrogel has become one of the most important hydrogel systems. A liquid formation in most cases provides an easier application however transformation to a solid gel increases the potential time in situ further leveraging the sustained release properties [14]. In addition to in situ hydrogel, contact lenses with high bioavailability and collagen shields with high biocompatibility have also frequently been investigated as ocular drug delivery systems and will be discussed in the following sections.

2.1 In Situ Hydrogels

One of the most important types of hydrogels is in situ hydrogels. In situ gelling systems are stimuli-responsive hydrogels, which can be applied to the eye as liquid and then mechanically transformed into gels. The in situ reversible hydrogels can swell, or de-swell based on the change in ion concentration, temperature or pH. All these types of stimuli-responsive hydrogels have been widely researched in ophthalmology.

Since in situ hydrogel exists in liquid form prior to mechanical transformation, it has been applied as a topical instillation on the corneal surface or injection into intraocular tissues, as discussed, the transformation leads to a significant increase in precorneal drug contact time, and consequently, an increase in bioavailability [14]. A combination of polyacrylic acid (Carbopol® 980NF) and hydroxypropyl methylcellulose (Methocel® K100LV) was utilized to prepare a pH-triggered hydrogel system for delivering ciprofloxacin [14]. To prevent any potential incompatibility between the drug and polyacrylic acid, ciprofloxacin was complexed with an ion exchange resin. The optimized product sustained drug delivery for 24 h in vitro, although the release kinetics followed a zero-order pattern for only up to 10 h. Important for both application and sustainability, it can maintain its stability for 3 months without any changes in clarity, drug content, pH, or gelling ability.

Moreover, in a rabbit model, no irritation was observed upon application of this in-situ hydrogel.

The injectable in situ hydrogels are especially appealing to be adapted in posterior eye diseases through intravitreal injection as liquid and transformed into solid form in vivo. This process serves to not only minimize the invasive effect but will prolong the time required for the drug to be released. Lai et al. developed an in situ hydrogel delivery system by utilizing gelatin grafted with carboxylic end-capped poly(*N*-isopropylacrylamide) to administer pilocarpine for glaucoma treatment [15]. The hydrogel underwent a phase transition from 25 to 34 °C and exhibited a cumulative drug release over 14 days, with an initial burst release in the first 30 min. In a rabbit model, the hydrogel was administered intracamerally and showed excellent bioadhesion, no inflammatory response, and degradation by MMP-2 over time. The hydrogel showed three times higher drug concentration in the aqueous humor compared to eye drop instillation after 4 h of treatment, indicating higher bioavailability. This represents a potential tangible difference with practical benefits to the patient and the treatment of the ocular condition.

2.2 Contact Lenses

The contact lens has also been proposed as a drug delivery system showing significantly improved bioavailability than topical formulations. Contact lens delivery systems achieve an extended residence time of more than 30 min, which is significantly higher than the normal residence time of only 1–3 min in eye drop delivery [2]. As expected, the longer residence time increased the drug bioavailability by up to 50%, suggesting the possibility of less frequent therapy, leading to higher patient compliance and potentially a faster healing process [2]. Against this, contact lens insertion will often require trained personnel for application. In 2022, FDA approved the first drug-eluting contact lenses, the ACUVUE® Theravision™ made of etafilcon A with ketotifen to prevent the itched eye induced by allergic conjunctivitis and correction of refractive ametropia [16]. Every lens contains 19 mcg of ketotifen, however, the process for how ketotifen combined with etafilcon A remains proprietary. Containing almost 2/3 water content (59%), it is expected to have an excellent safety profile [16]. Wetting agents such as polyvinylpyrrolidone are used in Etafilcon A lenses to mimic natural tear films and further improve comfort through both initial and extended wear [17]. Its clinical study showed less than 2% of participants experienced eye irritation or pain as a result of the procedure [17]. This initial product validated the promising effect of using contact lenses as a drug delivery system. This section will discuss various novel designs for encapsulating drugs in therapeutic contact lenses.

2.2.1 Soaking Method

The soaking method is the most simple and cost-effective way to encapsulate drugs in contact lenses. The contact lens has internal cavities/channels that can accommodate drug molecules. The drug reservoir ability is strongly dependent on the hydrophilic/hydrophobic components of contact lenses, the thickness of contact lenses, the molecular weight of drugs, the soaking time, and the concentration of drugs [2]. However, for most ophthalmic drugs, the contact lens has a low affinity, resulting in poor retention and burst release of drug encapsulated through the soaking method [2]. In an experiment of drug release following soaking in contact lenses, ophthalmic drugs including cromolyn sodium, ketorolac tromethamine, and dexamethasone sodium phosphate showed a quick release of less than 1 h, and ketotifen fumarate displayed a slower release of approximately 5 h [10]. For drugs including dexamethasone sodium phosphate, ketorolac tromethamine, and ketotifen fumarate, higher uptake was observed in materials with higher water content and higher pHEMA composition suggesting continued variability [10].

Several techniques have been developed to increase the drug loading efficacy of the soaking method and to achieve sustained and controlled drug delivery. Ryan et al. developed a rapid drug loading method for the hydrophobic drug latanoprost for only 4 min by soaking the drugs in *n*-propanol [18]. The amount of drug loading remains controllable and can reach up to 450ug per lens, and the drug release was proportional to the drug-loaded with a duration of up to 4 days. Cyclodextrin's structure consists of a hydrophilic outer surface and a hydrophobic cavity, which can form inclusion complexes with a variety of hydrophobic molecules. This property makes it particularly effective in delivering hydrophobic drugs [13]. To enhance the uptake of puerarin and achieve controlled and sustained release of the drug, β-cyclodextrin (β-CD) was encapsulated in pHEMA hydrogel [13]. When tested in a rabbit trial, the drug-eluted pHEMA lens with β-CD showed a higher average drug residence time of over 100 min compared with the drug-eluted pHEMA lens (81 ± 11 mins) and the 1% puerarin topical eye solution (13 ± 7 mins). Although the optimal balance remains to be elucidated, it would appear higher β-CD content would be more appropriate for success with a slower drug release.

2.2.2 Molecular Imprinting

Molecular imprinting refers to a technique using functional monomers imprinted to create artificial recognition sites in contact lenses, which can tailor the drug loading and release pattern (Fig. 3) [2]. The molecularly imprinted polymers are generated by free-radical polymerization, which involves the interaction between functional monomers and the target drug [19]. After polymerization, the target drug was removed from the imprinted material, leaving behind specific cavities that are complementary to the size and shape of the target drug. Macromolecular memory in contact lenses results in extended drug release over weeks [19, 20].

Negin et al. developed HEMA contact lenses for delivering antimicrobial peptides polymyxin B and vancomycin using the molecular imprinting method [20]. Acrylic acid-functionalization with imprinting increased the affinity of polymyxin B and vancomycin more than ten-fold on lenses, while nearly no uptake was observed in non-imprinted lenses. This affinity is proportional to the percentage of template molecules on lenses. In acrylic acid-imprinted lenses, both polymyxin B and vancomycin were released over a 2-week period, whereas in non-imprinted

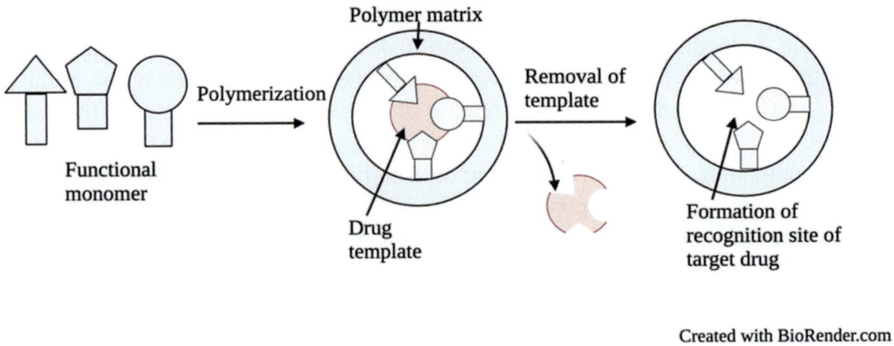

Fig. 3 The illustration of molecular imprinting drug loading method

lenses, the drug is released within a few hours. A recent study used molecular imprinting to deliver multiple drugs simultaneously. Diclofenac sodium (DS) and dexamethasone sodium phosphate (DMSP) or bromfenac sodium (BS) and moxifloxacin (MOX) were molecularly imprinted to contact lens [19]. Both DS + DMSP-loaded lenses and BS + MOX-loaded lenses showed sustained release of loaded drugs over 1 week. The stability of the mesh size before and after molecular imprinting confirms that the controlled release is attributed to macromolecular memory rather than a tighter structure or smaller mesh size.

2.2.3 Other Techniques

Other methods have been developed to enhance the drug's absorption and to achieve a sustained release of the drug from the contact lens. Supercritical fluid technology dissolves the drug in supercritical fluid and diffuses it into contact lenses, showing high loading efficiency. Supercritical fluids represent fluids whose temperature and pressure are greater than their critical temperature and critical pressure, allowing them to assume the properties of both a liquid and a gas. CO_2 is commonly used as a solvent in this technique due to its non-toxicity, high diffusivity, and low surface tension [21]. However, the cost of supercritical fluid technology is high. Furthermore, the drug loading and release behavior is strongly influenced by the operating conditions, such as temperature, pressure, and depressurization during drug impregnation, resulting in poor reproducibility [21]. The drug-loaded film coating for contact lenses has also been developed. To achieve the zero-order kinetics of drug delivery, Ciolino et al. created the drug-polymer film by mixing ciprofloxacin and PLGA (poly[lactic-*co*-glycolic acid]) (PLGA) polymer using the solvent casting method, followed by film coating on pHEMA contact lenses using ultraviolet (UV) polymerization [22]. The drug-polymer-coated lenses showed a sustained drug release with zero-order kinetics over 4 weeks. The increased barrier of drug diffusion was found in film with a higher ratio PLGA: drug ratio. The use of supercritical fluid technology and drug-loaded film coating is rapidly expanding and represents an option for drug delivery across numerous biomedical applications.

2.3 Collagen Shield

With high biocompatibility and biodegradability, collagen shield has also been explored as an ocular drug delivery system [23]. The collagen shield usually contains type I and type III collagen and is reserved in dehydrated form, which needs to be rehydrated before use [23]. The FDA has approved several collagen shields on the market, including Biocora®, MediLens®, and ProShield®, but there is no clear information about their composition or patient feedback. Collagen shields usually start to dissolve after 12, 24, and 72 h [23]. After the designed dissolution period, the collagen shield will lose 1/2 to 1/3 of its mass. By this point, its geometry will have changed, and it will become loose on the surface of the eye, allowing it to be easily removed.

Collagen shields can increase the drug contact time and maintain the concentration by serving as a reservoir and gradually releasing the drug as the shield dissolved [24]. Collagen shield has shown comparable or superior ability in the delivery in rabbit models of many antibiotics including vancomycin, gentamicin, tobramycin, and prednisolone acetate [25]. A 12-h collagen shield was soaked in prednisolone acetate for 15 mins prior to application in rabbit eyes. As compared to topical application, the drug concentration levels in the aqueous and cornea were 4–5 times higher after 30 mins and 100–200 times higher after 120 min [24]. Another study evaluated the drug delivery of dexamethasone with a 24-h collagen shield in both the anterior and posterior segments of rabbit eyes [25]. Compared with the single drop instillation, a 2–5-fold higher drug level was observed in the 20-min pre-soaked shield in the cornea, aqueous, iris, and vitreous over a 6-h period. This study further compared the treatment of hourly eye drop alone to a pre-soaked collagen shield plus hourly eye drop. The results showed collagen shields with supplementary hourly eye drops can maintain twofold higher drug levels in the cornea, aqueous, iris, and vitreous compared with hourly eye drops alone over 6 h highlighting a significant potential additive impact. Despite the collagen shield's advantages over topical eye drops, it is limited by its requirement of professional installation [23]. Similar to contact lenses, the burst release phenomenon still exists in the collagen shield drug delivery [26]. Furthermore, although the collagen shield has high tolerance with regard to comfort in the eye, it has low transparency, resulting in a reduction in visual acuity to 6/36–6/60 [23]. Although there are some collagen shields have been approved by FDA, they are still not frequently used in the clinic.

3 Nanosystems

The use of nanosystems in drug delivery has attracted increasing attention to enhance the penetration of ophthalmic drugs and prolong drug release. They also showed benefits to protecting the unstable drug from premature degradation by inhibiting the premature interaction of the drug with the biological environment [27]. Nanosystems can actively incorporate into cell membranes via different endocytic pathways and can be used to deliver poorly permeable small molecules and proteins [28]. In general, nanocarriers with smaller sizes remain preferred because of lower irritation and better bioavailability [27]. Several factors affect the mechanism of drug release from these nanocarriers, including the stability of the carrier, drug–carrier interaction, and drug diffusion [27]. A variety of nanocarriers have been studied for use as ocular drug delivery systems. The three most widely studied nanocarriers are liposomes, dendrimers, and polymeric nanoparticles including nanospheres and nanocapsules.

3.1 Liposome

The liposome is a spherical vehicle made of a double layer of phospholipids with an aqueous core (Fig. 4). Liposomes can have single or multiple phospholipids double layers, resulting in a wide size range from 10 nm to 1 μm [29]. It is a biodegradable and biocompatible carrier for both hydrophilic and hydrophobic drugs [29]. Hydrophilic drugs can be encapsulated in the aqueous core and hydrophobic drugs can be encapsulated in the lipid membrane (Fig. 4).

The use of liposomes in ocular drug delivery has been demonstrated by several researchers in the last few decades, and some liposomal drugs are currently available in clinics. For example, Visudyne®, a liposomal intravenous drug system has been approved by FDA and utilized successfully for many years for treating choroidal neovascularization caused by macular degeneration, pathologic myopia, and ocular histoplasmosis.

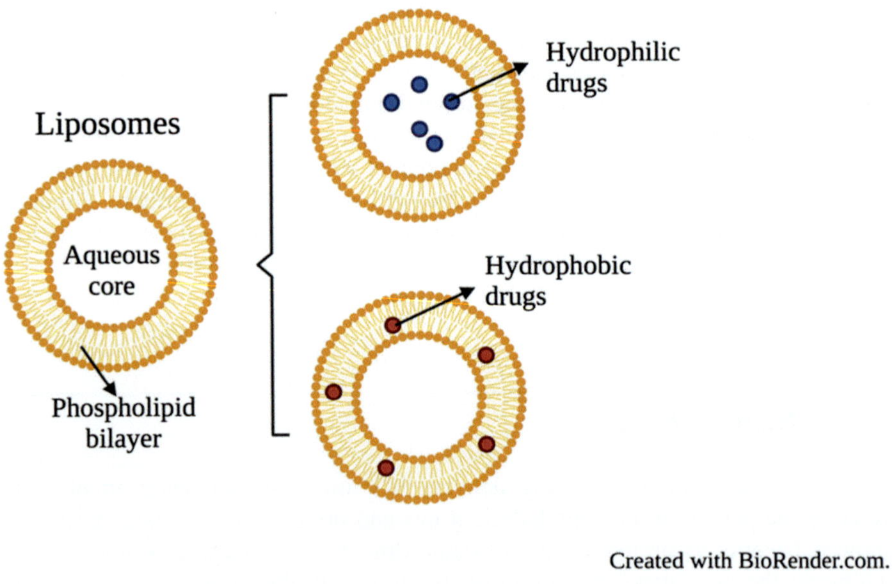

Fig. 4 Structure of liposomes for drug delivery application

Drugs in the liposomal formulation have shown higher biocompatibility than commercial eye drop formulation [30]. Different materials have been explored to improve the mucoadhesive property of liposomes. It is reported that positively charged liposomes have higher affinity on the ocular surface compared with negatively charged or neutral liposomes because they can bind to negative-charged mucin on the corneal epithelium [29]. In a rabbit model, dioctadecyldimethylammonium bromide *(DODAB)* and stearyl amine (SA) have been used as positive charge-inducing agents to generate cationic liposomal ciprofloxacin, which has shown more than threefold higher bioavailability compared with commercially available eye drops [31]. Coating bioadhesive polymers such as chitosan and carbomer can also be used to modify liposomes for mucoadhesive properties. Carbomer with good bioadhesive properties and good ocular tolerability has also been used to synthesize carbomer-coated liposomal ciprofloxacin [29]. The in vivo drug-releasing test in rabbit eyes showed an approximately fourfold higher bioavailability in the carbomer-coated liposome formulation compared with the commercial ciprofloxacin eye drop [29]. To improve the mucoadhesive property, it is preferable to coat liposomes with natural polymers rather than using charge-inducing chemicals like SA and DODAB due to their potential cytotoxicity. Furthermore, it has been demonstrated that polymeric liposomes coated with natural polymers, such as chitosan, even if charged negatively with dicetylphosphate (DP), are more mucoadhesive than liposomes that have been cationized with SA [30].

3.2 Dendrimers

Dendrimers are nanovehicles made of high-branching "tree-like" structured polymers with well-defined shapes and sizes [27].The shape of dendrimers consists of a central core and "radically concentric layers" known as "generations" (Fig. 5). Dendrimer has extraordinary structure control of linear increase in diameter with the increase in generation [32].While many dendrimer families have been synthesized, polyamidoamine (PAMAM) dendrimer is the most widely studied. In PAMAM dendrimers, ammonia or ethylenediamine core binds with the amine groups of branches and amides [32].

Dendrimers can deliver lipophilic drugs through direct encapsulation in the inner oily cavity. It can carry hydrophilic drugs by bonding them on the surface through covalent or electrostatic interaction [32]. There are also terminal groups in dendrimers that can be employed to make drug-dendrimer conjugation. For example, DenTimol developed to treat glaucoma was synthesized by conjugating timolol in PAMAM G3 dendrimer surface through the polyethylene glycol (PEG) terminal group [33]. This system shows increased efficiency in penetrating the cornea, leading to a quick reduction of an important risk factor, elevated intraocular pressure (IOP), by 30% in less than 30 min in rabbit eyes [33]. However, dendrimers have raised concerns due to their potential cytotoxicity. Scientists have demonstrated that the cytotoxicity of dendrimers is highly linked with the generations and properties

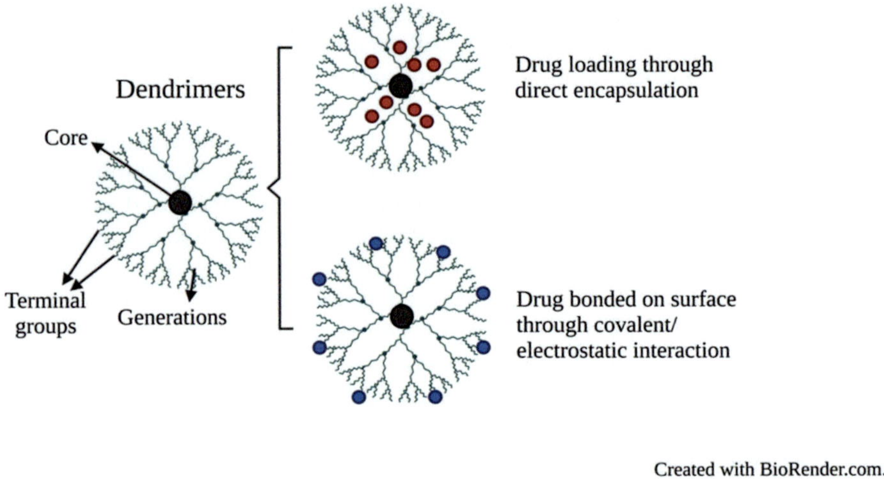

Fig. 5 Structure of dendrimer for drug delivery application

of terminal groups [34]. In general, those dendrimers with higher generation and positive charges on their surface exhibited greater cytotoxicity [34].

3.3 Polymeric Nanoparticles

Polymeric nanoparticles can be made of biodegradable natural polymers including alginate, chitosan, gelatin, and albumin, or synthetic polymers including poly(lactide) (PLA), poly(lactide-*co*-glycolide) (PLGA), and poly (ε-caprolactone) (PCL) [35]. Biodegradable nanoparticles are frequently utilized due to their higher biocompatibility. Nanoparticles are divided into two main categories based on the inner structure: nanosphere and nanocapsule (Fig. 6) [35]. Nanosphere, ranging in size from 100 to 1000 nm, is defined as a matrix system, in which the drug is dispersed evenly in the matrix or is absorbed on the surface (Fig. 6a). The nanocapsule, ranging in size from 10 to 1000 nm, is composed of a hydrophobic core and polymeric envelope, in which the hydrophobic drug can be entrapped into the cavity or absorbed on the surface (Fig. 6b).

Polymeric nanoparticles have been extensively studied to improve drug contact time and increase bioavailability. A nanoparticle consisting of two polymers, namely mucoadhesive hyaluronic acid and biocompatible zein, has been synthesized to enhance the bioavailability and stability of ciprofloxacin [36]. The polymeric nanoparticle system exhibited an initial burst release followed by a sustained release over 24 h while maintaining high biocompatibility and encapsulation efficiency. Positively charged polymeric nanoparticles have demonstrated enhanced drug delivery properties due to their bioadhesive nature to negatively charged ocular surfaces [12]. Cationic nanoparticles composed of Eudragit RLPO® polymer were employed to deliver the antifungal drug terconazole (TCZ), which

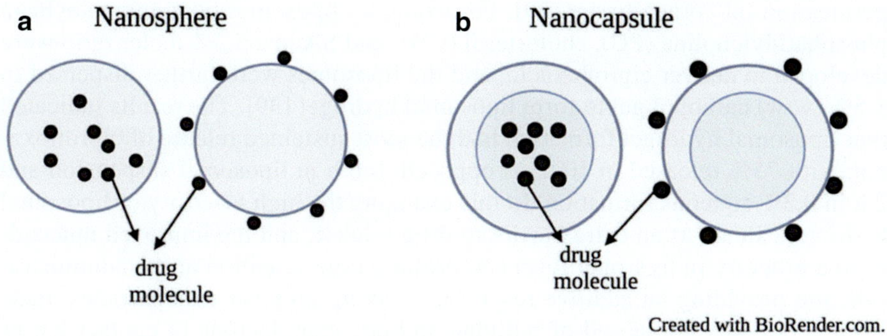

Fig. 6 Structure of (**a**) nanosphere and (**b**) nanocapsule for drug delivery application

exhibited mucoadhesive properties and sustained drug delivery over 24 h in vitro and a 2.3-fold higher antimycotic activity compared with plain TCZ solution [12]. However, despite the demonstrated effectiveness of these polymeric nanoparticles in drug delivery, potential cytotoxicity resulting from the release of toxic monomers during degradation and residual material associated with them remains a concern [37].

4 Comparison of the Delivery of Ciprofloxacin in Different Systems

Ciprofloxacin is used as a case to discuss the differences between various drug delivery systems. The fluoroquinolone antibiotic ciprofloxacin has a broad use in both Gram-positive and Gram-negative bacterial infections [38]. This hydrophilic drug has been widely explored in a variety of novel drug carriers including contact lenses, in situ hydrogel, liposomes, and polymeric nanoparticles, to achieve sustained and controlled drug delivery with zero-order kinetics. In the application of all these carriers, longer ciprofloxacin contact time and higher biocompatibility have been achieved when compared with commercial eye drop instillation. Polymeric nanoparticles, liposomes, and in situ hydrogel showed 8–24 h of ciprofloxacin releasing, with burst releasing remaining a challenge in these systems [14, 30, 36]. Contact lens soaking in the ciprofloxacin showed quick release in a few hours. However, when other techniques including molecular imprinting were employed, it showed extended releasing time, even over weeks representing a significant potential clinical advantage [19, 20].

Sustained drug delivery can be achieved when these techniques were used in combination. Nanocarriers, because of their small size, are usually investigated to be encapsulated in other macro-sized carriers such as hydrogel and contact lenses for sustained drug delivery and have shown improved efficacy in drug delivery. Compared with liposomes alone, the liposome in hydrogel form showed retarded and more extended ciprofloxacin release as well as higher drug permeation on cornea tissue [39]. For example, liposomes containing soybean phosphatidylcholine (PC), cholesterol (CH), and SA in a 5:3:1 molar ratio were developed to deliver ciprofloxacin, and the liposomes were further dispersed in 1.5% (w/w) carbopol gel to form liposomal hydrogel [39]. The results indicated that liposomal hydrogel formation had the most sustained release of ciprofloxacin, with 75% released in 10 h, as opposed to 6 h in liposomal suspension and 2 h in 0.3% aqueous formation. In this example, the high viscosity of liposomal hydrogel can act as an extra barrier to drug release, and the improved mucoadhesive property in hydrogel form can prolong drug retention at the administration site providing an additive response. Soaking polymer nanoparticles made from copolymer composed of pullulan and polycaprolactone in contact lenses also showed sustained ciprofloxacin release over 24 h, with a concentration higher than the minimal inhibition concentration of *S. aureus* and *P. aeruginosa* [38]. In addition, it has been shown that drug release behavior is affected not only by the properties of drug carriers but also by drug release systems. Drug release systems in a physiological flow exhibit a slower and more consistent release rate than in a vial system [40]. In fixed-volume vials, the release of ciprofloxacin from contact lenses typically takes approximately 2 h, whereas under physiological flow conditions, a gradual and steady release of the drug over 24 h was observed [40].

5 Discussion and Conclusion

Improving the efficacy of drug delivery in the ocular system is a long-standing challenge. The topical administration has many limitations, especially the low bioavailability and short drug contact time. Novel alternative drug delivery systems have been generated to overcome these limitations including using hydrogel and nanocarrier systems. These techniques have also been used individually or combined for a more sustained and controlled drug release, resulting in a reduced dose frequency and leading to potentially higher patient compliance. A number of these techniques have been approved by FDA and are currently available in the clinic, including the most recently approved drug-eluting contact lens ACUVUE Theravision by FDA in 2022. These successes indicate the promising direction in using hydrogel and nanocarriers as alternatives to topical eye drops. However, challenges including the burst release still need to be addressed. Furthermore, more research needs to be carried out on the potential cytotoxicity of nanocarriers in ocular drug delivery and the clinical impact on the patient. Research interests also focus on other factors such as drug loading efficiency and drug penetration efficiency to improve bioavailability. Combining nanocarriers and hydrogel systems has demonstrated increased drug contact time and higher bioavailability when compared to drug delivery with either nanocarriers or hydrogel alone. Therefore, this approach holds significant potential for further investigation.

References

1. Gaudana R, Ananthula HK, Parenky A, Mitra AK. Ocular drug delivery. AAPS J. 2010;12:348–60.
2. Maulvi FA, Soni TG, Shah DO. A review on therapeutic contact lenses for ocular drug delivery. Drug Deliv. 2016;23:3017–26.
3. Agrahari V, et al. A comprehensive insight on ocular pharmacokinetics. Drug Deliv Transl Res. 2016;6:735–54.
4. Huang A, Tseng S, Kenyon K. Paracellular permeability of corneal and conjunctival epithelia. Invest Ophthalmol Vis Sci. 1989;30:684–9.
5. Gokhale NS. Medical management approach to infectious keratitis. Indian J Ophthalmol. 2008;56:215–20.
6. Li J, Mooney DJ. Designing hydrogels for controlled drug delivery. Nat Rev Mater. 2016;1:16071.
7. Lynch CR, et al. Hydrogel biomaterials for application in ocular drug delivery. Front Bioeng Biotechnol. 2020;8:228.
8. Bhattarai N, Gunn J, Zhang M. Chitosan-based hydrogels for controlled, localized drug delivery. Adv Drug Deliv Rev. 2010;62:83–99.
9. Hezaveh H, Muhamad II. Controlled drug release via minimization of burst release in pH-response kappa-carrageenan/polyvinyl alcohol hydrogels. Chem Eng Res Des. 2013;91:508–19.
10. Karlgard CCS, Wong NS, Jones LW, Moresoli C. In vitro uptake and release studies of ocular pharmaceutical agents by silicon-containing and p-HEMA hydrogel contact lens materials. Int J Pharm. 2003;257:141–51.
11. Huang X, Brazel CS. Analysis of burst release of proxyphylline from poly(vinyl alcohol) hydrogels. Chem Eng Commun. 2003;190:519–32.
12. Mohsen AM. Cationic polymeric nanoparticles for improved ocular delivery and antimycotic activity of terconazole. J Pharm Sci. 2022;111:458–68.
13. Xu J, Li X, Sun F. Cyclodextrin-containing hydrogels for contact lenses as a platform for drug incorporation and release. Acta Biomater. 2010;6:486–93.
14. Jain SP, Shah SP, Rajadhyaksha NS, Singh PSP, Amin PD. In situ ophthalmic gel of ciprofloxacin hydrochloride for once a day sustained delivery. Drug Dev Ind Pharm. 2008;34:445–52.
15. Lai JY, Hsieh AC. A gelatin-g-poly(N-isopropylacrylamide) biodegradable in situ gelling delivery system for the intracameral administration of pilocarpine. Biomaterials. 2012;33:2372–87.
16. FDA (US Food and Drug Administration). Highlights of prescribing information ACUVUE® Theravision™ with Ketotifen. Food and Drug Administration Web site. https://www.accessdata.fda.gov/drugsatfda_docs/label/2022/022388s000lbl.pdf. Accessed 2022.
17. Miller J, Giedd B, Subbaraman LN. Clinical comparison of a silicone hydrogel and a conventional hydrogel daily disposable contact lens. Clin Ophthalmol. 2021;15:4339–45.
18. Horne RR, Rich JT, Bradley MW, Pitt WG. Latanoprost uptake and release from commercial contact lenses. J Biomater Sci Polym Ed. 2020;31:1–19.
19. DiPasquale SA, Uricoli B, DiCerbo MC, Brown TL, Byrne ME. Controlled release of multiple therapeutics from silicone hydrogel contact lenses for post-cataract/post-refractive surgery and uveitis treatment. Transl Vis Sci Technol. 2021;10:5.
20. Malakooti N, Alexander C, Alvarez-Lorenzo C. Imprinted contact lenses for sustained release of polymyxin B and related antimicrobial peptides. J Pharm Sci. 2015;104:3386–94.
21. Yokozaki Y, Sakabe J, Ng B, Shimoyama Y. Effect of temperature, pressure and depressurization rate on release profile of salicylic acid from contact lenses prepared by supercritical carbon dioxide impregnation. Chem Eng Res Des. 2015;100:89–94.
22. Ciolino JB, et al. A drug-eluting contact lens. Invest Ophthalmol Vis Sci. 2009;50:3346–52.
23. Willoughby CE, Batterbury M, Kaye SB. Collagen corneal shields. Surv Ophthalmol. 2002;47:174–82.
24. Sawusch MR, O'Brien TP, Updegraff SA. Collagen corneal shields enhance penetration of topical prednisolone acetate. J Cataract Refract Surg. 1989;15:625–8.

25. Hwang DG, Stern WH, Hwang PH, MacGowan-Smith LA. Collagen shield enhancement of topical dexamethasone penetration. Arch Ophthalmol. 1989;107:1375–80.
26. Zhou S, et al. Release of moxifloxacin from corneal collagen shields. Eye Contact Lens. 2018;44(Suppl 2):S143–s147.
27. Omerović N, Vranić E. Application of nanoparticles in ocular drug delivery systems. Heal Technol. 2020;10:61–78.
28. Mosquera J, García I, Liz-Marzán LM. Cellular uptake of nanoparticles versus small molecules: a matter of size. Acc Chem Res. 2018;51:2305–13.
29. Feghhi M, Sharif Makhmalzadeh B, Farrahi F, Akmali M, Hasanvand N. Anti-microbial effect and in vivo ocular delivery of ciprofloxacin-loaded liposome through Rabbit's eye. Curr Eye Res. 2020;45:1245–51.
30. Abdelbary G. Ocular ciprofloxacin hydrochloride mucoadhesive chitosan-coated liposomes. Pharm Dev Technol. 2011;16:44–56.
31. Taha EI, El-Anazi MH, El-Bagory IM, Bayomi MA. Design of liposomal colloidal systems for ocular delivery of ciprofloxacin. Saudi Pharm J. 2014;22:231–9.
32. Esfand R, Tomalia DA. Poly(amidoamine) (PAMAM) dendrimers: from biomimicry to drug delivery and biomedical applications. Drug Discov Today. 2001;6:427–36.
33. Lancina MG 3rd, Wang J, Williamson GS, Yang H. DenTimol as a Dendrimeric timolol analogue for glaucoma therapy: synthesis and preliminary efficacy and safety assessment. Mol Pharm. 2018;15:2883–9.
34. Janaszewska A, Lazniewska J, Trzepiński P, Marcinkowska M, Klajnert-Maculewicz B. Cytotoxicity of dendrimers. Biomol Ther. 2019;9(8):330.
35. Franco P, De Marco I. Contact lenses as ophthalmic drug delivery systems: a review. Polymers (Basel). 2021;13:1102.
36. Jacinto TA, Oliveira B, Miguel SP, Ribeiro MP, Coutinho P. Ciprofloxacin-loaded zein/hyaluronic acid nanoparticles for ocular mucosa delivery. Pharmaceutics. 2022;14:1557.
37. Sharma S, Parveen R, Chatterji BP. Toxicology of nanoparticles in drug delivery. Curr Pathobiol Rep. 2021;9:133–44.
38. Garhwal R, et al. Sustained ocular delivery of ciprofloxacin using nanospheres and conventional contact lens materials. Invest Ophthalmol Vis Sci. 2012;53:1341–52.
39. Hosny KM. Ciprofloxacin as ocular liposomal hydrogel. AAPS PharmSciTech. 2010;11:241–6.
40. Bajgrowicz M, Phan CM, Subbaraman LN, Jones L. Release of ciprofloxacin and moxifloxacin from daily disposable contact lenses from an in vitro eye model. Invest Ophthalmol Vis Sci. 2015;56:2234–42.

Clinical Trials Relevant for Optometrists

Parul Ichhpujani and Surbhi Kapoor

The landmark clinical trials in Ophthalmology provide an inside look at the therapeutic pipeline and how the standardized treatment protocols can objectively guide patient care, which strategies to adopt and which to discontinue. This chapter enlists a few landmark clinical trials which may help optometry practitioners and students to uncover better ways to prevent, diagnose, treat, and understand common ophthalmic disorders. For ease of the readers, the trial results and conclusions have been tabulated.

1 Pediatric Eye Disease Investigator Group (PEDIG)

Amblyopia, or lazy eye, refers to a unilateral or bilateral decrease of vision, caused by abnormal vision development in infancy or childhood. It is the leading cause of decreased vision among children.

Spectacle correction with occlusion or penalization therapy using atropine eye drops is generally considered the first treatment options for amblyopia. Clinically effective health care requires informed decisions based on evidence-based treatment. Over- or underutilization of the prescribed therapy often leads to poor visual recovery [1]. For children with amblyopia, evidence-based treatment has been made possible by the landmark Pediatric Eye Disease Investigator Group (PEDIG) research. This study compared the result of patching and atropine as treatments for moderate amblyopia in children younger than 7 years [2].

P. Ichhpujani (✉) · S. Kapoor
Department of Ophthalmology, Government Medical College and Hospital, Chandigarh, India

D. Shu et al. (eds.), *Current Advances in Optometry*, Current Practices in Ophthalmology, https://doi.org/10.1007/978-981-97-8140-9_10

Disease entity	Study group	Results	Conclusion
Amblyopia with visual acuity from 20/40 to 20/100 * 419 patients (3–7 years old) * 507 patients (7–17 years old)	**3–7 years old group:** 1. Patching 2. Atropine **7–17 years old group:** 1. Patching + atropine 2. Optical correction alone	**3–7 years old group:** Visual acuity improvement: 3.16 in patching group vs. 2.84 in atropine group **7–17 years old group:** Patching and near vision exercise can improve visual acuity from 7 to 12 years even if previously treated. This is less effective for the 13–17 years age group	Atropine and patching produce improvement of similar magnitude, and both are appropriate modalities for the initial treatment of moderate amblyopia in children aged 3 to <7 years. For kids 7–12 years old, a combined program of patching and near vision exercise can improve visual acuity. This is less effective in age 13–17 year olds

2 Infant Aphakia Treatment Study (IATS)

Unilateral congenital cataracts lead to deprivation amblyopia, which can be severe, unless early surgical intervention is done [3]. The answer as regards the best type of optical correction for the monocular aphakia resulting from cataract extraction came from IATS. This study compared the visual outcomes and adverse events of contact lens (CL) to primary intraocular lens (IOL) correction of monocular aphakia during infancy.

IATS found that good visual acuity and stereopsis could be achieved in some patients in both the CL and IOL groups. Early cataract surgery, appropriate optical correction, and part-time occlusion of the fellow eye are important to achieve good vision [4]. However, excessive occlusion of the fellow eye may disrupt the development of stereopsis. Additionally, IOL implantation may be associated with adverse effects such as the visual axis opacification. A 10-year follow-up study showed that glaucoma-related adverse events occurred in 40% of eyes, unrelated to IOL implantation. More research is needed to provide a perfect visual outcome for these children.

Disease entity	Study group	Results	Conclusion
• Unilateral congenital cataract undergoing cataract surgery between 1 and 6 months of age • 114 patients	Group 1: IOL implantation Group 2: CL correction	Median logMAR: 0.80 in CL group vs. 0.97 in IOL group ($p = 0.20$) Additional surgeries: 12% in CL group vs. 63% in IOL group	Caution should be exercised when performing IOL implantation in children 6 months of age or younger given the higher incidence of adverse events and the absence of an improved short-term visual outcome compared to CL use

3 Low-Concentration Atropine for Myopia Progression (LAMP) Study

Most infants are born hyperopic, and their hyperopia reduces as the eyeball elongates alongwith flattening of cornea. Both genetic and environmental factors influence the onset and progression of myopia. Increased near work, less outdoor activities, and lifestyle ruled by smartphones/tablets are responsible for the early development of myopia at a younger age. The prevalence rate of myopia is increasing worldwide, and as per WHO, it is projected to increase to 52% by 2050 [5]. The available treatment options for the control of myopia include spectacle correction, contact lenses, keratorefractive surgery, and pharmaceuticals agents such as low dose atropine. However, there are no perfect therapeutic modalities that effectively halt and slow down the development of myopia without causing significant side effects.

LAMP study evaluated the efficacy and safety of low-concentration atropine eye drops at 0.05%, 0.025%, and 0.01% compared with placebo over a 1-year period. [6] The study was a double-blinded, randomized, and placebo-controlled therefore it provided robust evidence. It has delineated a concentration-dependent response, both as regards efficacy and side effect profile in the low-atropine concentration range from 0.05% to 0.01%. Higher concentration of low-concentration atropine 0.05% is most efficacious among the three concentration.

The LAMP phase 2: In a follow-up study, over 2 years, the efficacy of 0.05% atropine observed was double that of 0.01% atropine, and it remained the optimal concentration among the studied atropine concentrations in slowing myopia progression [7].

Disease entity	Study group	Results	Conclusion
438 children aged 4–12 years. with myopia of at least −1.0 diopter (D) and astigmatism of −2.5 D or less	Randomly assigned in a 1:1:1:1 ratio to receive 0.05%, 0.025%, and 0.01% atropine eye drops, or placebo eye drop, respectively, once at bedtime to both eyes for 1 year	* After 1 year, the mean SE change was significant($P < 0.001$) in the 0.05%, 0.025%, and 0.01% atropine groups, and placebo groups, with a significant ($P < 0.001$) mean increase in AL * Accommodation amplitude was also significantly reduced ($P < 0.001$)	* The 0.05%, 0.025%, and 0.01% atropine drops reduced myopia progression along a concentration-dependent response * Of the three concentrations, 0.05% atropine was most effective in controlling SE progression and AL elongation over a period of 1 year

4 Atropine for the Treatment of Myopia 1 (ATOM 1)

The ATOM 1 study was a randomized, placebo-controlled trial designed to assess the safety and efficacy of topical atropine in controlling the progression of myopia in children [8].

Disease entity	Study group	Results	Conclusion
400 children aged 6–12 years with myopia of −1 D to −6 D and astigmatism of −1.50 D or less	* Randomly assigned with equal probability to receive either 1% atropine eye drop or Isoptotears once nightly * Followed-up at 4-monthly intervals for 2 years	* At 1 year, mean myopia progression in the placebo-control eyes was −0.76 D ± 0.44 D * In atropine-treated eyes, however, there was a regression of myopia by +0.3 D ± 0.50 D ($p < 0.0001$)	Atropine 1% helped in controlling childhood myopia progression and axial elongation

5 Atropine for the Treatment of Myopia 2 (ATOM 2)

ATOM 2 was carried out to compare efficacy and visual side effects of three lower doses of atropine: 0.5%, 0.1%, and 0.01%. [9]

Disease entity	Study group	Results	Conclusion
400 children aged 6–12 years with myopia of at least −2.0 D and astigmatism of −1.50 D or less	Randomly assigned in a 2:2:1 ratio to 0.5%, 0.1%, and 0.01% atropine to be administered once nightly to both eyes for 2 years	Mean myopia progression at 2 years was −0.30 ± 0.60, −0.38 ± 0.60, and −0.49 ± 0.63 D in the atropine 0.5%, 0.1%, and 0.01% groups, respectively ($P = 0.02$ between the 0.01 and 0.5% groups; between other concentrations ($P > 0.05$)	Atropine 0.01% has minimal side effects compared with atropine at 0.1 and 0.5%, and retains comparable efficacy in controlling myopia progression

A rebound phenomenon was seen following the cessation of atropine 1%, 0.5%, 0.1%, and 0.01%, in ATOM 1 and ATOM 2 studies.

LAMP phase 3 study plans to look more into the rebound phenomenon by randomizing each of the three groups 0.05%, 0.025%, and 0.01% into wash out group and treatment-continued group, to evaluate the efficacy of 0.05%, 0.025%, and 0.01% atropine group during 3 years; whether treatment should be stopped after 2 years of atropine.

6 Zhongshan Angle Closure Prevention (ZAP) Trial

Primary angle closure disease constitutes a spectrum that includes primary angle closure suspects (PACS), primary angle closure (PAC, occludable angles with signs suggestive of outflow obstruction in absence of glaucomatous optic neuropathy) and primary angle closure glaucoma (PACG; occludable angles with glaucomatous optic neuropathy).

Most practitioners routinely offer prophylactic laser peripheral iridotomies (LPI) to PAC and PACG patients and only to a select few PACS ones. The ZAP trial was conducted to assess the efficacy and safety of LPI prophylaxis for Chinese patients with PACS [10]. The study found that although the LPI is effective in preventing progression from PACS to PAC, given the low incidence of development of PAC both in untreated and treated groups, LPI is not mandatorily recommended in glaucoma screening programs. However, the low rates of progression of PACS could be unique to Chinese population and this must be kept in mind when making clinical decisions regarding LPI for patients with PACS.

Disease entity	Study group	Results	Conclusion
PACS defined as angle closure • ≥6 h • No PAS • IOP < 21	$n = 889$ Group 1 = Laser PI (in one eye) Group 2 = Observation (in other eye)	Incidence of PAC = 4.19/1000 eye years in treated eyes compared with 7.97/1000 eye years in untreated eyes	PAC occurred in significant more untreated eyes (30 vs. 19) mostly due to development of PAS

7 Ocular Hypertension Treatment Study 1

Ocular Hypertension (OHT) is defined as elevated intraocular pressure (IOP) more than 21 mmHg on two or more occasions in the presence of open angles with no glaucomatous optic neuropathy or visual field defects. OHT is a significant risk factor for development of primary open angle glaucoma, and it is imperative that these patients be considered as glaucoma suspects and kept under follow up.

The landmark OHTS can guide who to observe and who to treat [11]. The first goal of this study was to determine if early treatment of people with elevated intraocular pressure (IOP) with topical antiglaucoma medication, would prevent them from developing POAG. The second goal was to determine baseline clinical and demographic factors that predict which people were more likely to develop glaucoma, and benefit from treatment. The study found that the predictive factors for developing POAG included increasing age, elevated IOP, thin corneas, and increased cup/disc ratio.

Disease entity	Study group	Results	Conclusion
1636 ocular hypertensive participants	Group 1 = topical hypotensive eye drops Group 2 = observation	Cumulative probability of developing POAG was 4.4% in medication group and 9.5% in observation group at 60 months	Topical antiglaucoma medication was effective in preventing or delaying the onset of POAG in individuals with elevated IOP and associated risk factors such as black race, thin CCT, male gender

The conclusion was that some individuals with OHTN might benefit from receiving early treatment, whereas most others were at such low risk that they did not need antiglaucoma treatment.

8 Ocular Hypertension Treatment Study 2

Both of the original randomization groups received medication during the OHTS 2 [12]. In OHTS phase 2, participants previously randomized to treatment for a mean of 7.5 years remained on treatment for a mean of 5.5 additional years. The data was analyzed to determine if the cumulative incidence of POAG was greater in the delayed treatment group and if the subsequent course after diagnosis is worse in the delayed treatment group. OHTS 2 found that the incidence of POAG was generally equal in the two randomization groups (HR, 1.06).

Delaying treatment in the observation group during the OHTS 1 did not initiate a process of irreversible deterioration in most participants. Most OHT patients are at low risk could be followed at less frequent intervals without treatment.

Disease entity	Study group	Results	Conclusion
1636 ocular hypertensive participants from OHTS 1	1572 surviving participants; out of which 1385 were "active" participants	* Cumulative proportion of participants who developed POAG from randomization to 13 years of follow-up was 0.22 in original observation group and 0.16 in original medication group ($P = 0.009$) * Median time to develop POAG was 6 years in the observation group and 8.7 years in the medication group	* There is a modest penalty for delaying treatment in OHT subjects which is minimal for low risk patients and more substantial for high-risk patients * High-risk patients may benefit from more frequent examinations and from early treatment

9 Ocular Hypertension Treatment Study 3

The OHTS Phase 3 built up on the groundwork done by the previous two studies. It aimed to determine the incidence and severity of POAG in the cohort and develop a 20-year prediction model including the previous factors identified and potential new risk factors [13]. In the OHTS 3, more than 70% of patients were receiving topical ocular hypotensive treatment, and some patients had undergone glaucoma surgery. It was noted that only one-fourth of participants in the OHTS developed visual field loss in either eye over long-term follow-up. The cumulative incidence of POAG at 20 years, adjusted for exposure time, was 45.6%. The incidence of POAG appeared to be generally linear over 20 years, with a possible modest increase in the rate of conversion after 15 years. The study developed a model that identified slow versus fast visual field progressors.

10 Laser in Glaucoma and Ocular Hypertension (LiGHT) Trial

Not all OHT patients who need treatment for IOP control prefer antiglaucoma medications. Selective laser trabeculoplasty (SLT) could offer an efficacious and adverse effect free temporary solution. The answer came from the Laser in Glaucoma and Ocular Hypertension (LiGHT) Trial, which has shown that SLT is a cost-effective solution for both OAG and OHT at 3 years [14]. This trial reported that the health-related quality of life (HRQoL) and clinical effectiveness of initial treatment with SLT compared with IOP-lowering eye drops after 6 years of treatment.

Disease entity	Study group	Results	Conclusion
718 patients	Group 1 = SLT group Group 2 = antiglaucoma drops	* 652 (91%) returned the primary outcome questionnaire at 36 month * Average EQ-5 D score: SLT: 0.89; eye drops: 0.90	SLT is a safe treatment for OAG and OHT, providing better long-term disease control than initial drop therapy, with reduced need for incisional glaucoma and cataract surgery over 6 years

References

1. Holmes JM, Beck RW, Kraker RT, et al. Pediatric Eye Disease Investigator Group. Risk of amblyopia recurrence after cessation of treatment. J AAPOS. 2004;8(5):420–8.
2. Repka MX, Beck RW, Holmes JM, et al. Pediatric Eye Disease Investigator Group. A randomized trial of patching regimens for treatment of moderate amblyopia in children. Arch Ophthalmol. 2003;121(5):603–11.
3. Louison S, Blanc J, Pallot C, Alassane S, Praudel A, Bron AM, et al. Visual outcomes and complications of congenital cataract surgery. J Fr Ophtalmol. 2019;42(4):368–74.
4. Lenhart PD, Lambert SR. Current management of infantile cataracts. Surv Ophthalmol. 2022;67(5):1476–505.
5. Singh H, Singh H, Latief U, Tung GK, Shahtaghi NR, Sahajpal NS, Kaur I, Jain SK. Myopia, its prevalence, current therapeutic strategy and recent developments: a review. Indian J Ophthalmol. 2022;70(8):2788–99.

6. Yam JC, Jiang Y, Tang SM, Law AKP, et al. Low-concentration atropine for myopia progression (LAMP) study: a randomized, double-blinded, placebo-controlled trial of 0.05%, 0.025%, and 0.01% atropine eye drops in myopia control. Ophthalmology. 2019;126(1):113–24.
7. Yam JC, Li FF, Zhang X, Tang SM, et al. Two-year clinical trial of the low-concentration atropine for myopia progression (LAMP) study: phase 2 report. Ophthalmology. 2020;127(7):910–9.
8. Chua WH, Balakrishnan V, Chan YH, Tong L, Ling Y, Quah BL, Tan D. Atropine for the treatment of childhood myopia. Ophthalmology. 2006;113(12):2285–91.
9. Chia A, Chua WH, Cheung YB, Wong WL, Lingham A, Fong A, Tan D. Atropine for the treatment of childhood myopia: safety and efficacy of 0.5%, 0.1%, and 0.01% doses (atropine for the treatment of myopia 2). Ophthalmology. 2012;119(2):347–54.
10. Han JE, Myo A, Mathew RG, Henein C. Infographic: Zhongshan angle closure prevention (ZAP) trial. Eye (Lond). 2021;35(12):3185–6.
11. Gordon MO, Kass MA. What we have learned from the ocular hypertension treatment study. Am J Ophthalmol. 2018;189:xxiv–xxvii.
12. Gordon MO, Gao F, Beiser JA, Miller JP, Kass MA. The 10-year incidence of glaucoma among patients with treated and untreated ocular hypertension Arch Ophthalmol 2011;129(12):1630–1631.
13. Kass MA, Heuer DK, Higginbotham EJ, Parrish RK, Khanna CL, Brandt JD, Soltau JB, Johnson CA, Keltner JL, Huecker JB, Wilson BS, Liu L, Miller JP, Quigley HA, Gordon MO, Ocular Hypertension Study Group. Assessment of cumulative incidence and severity of primary open-angle glaucoma among participants in the ocular hypertension treatment study after 20 years of follow-up. JAMA Ophthalmol. 2021;139(5):1–9.
14. Gazzard G, Konstantakopoulou E, Garway-Heath D, Adeleke M, Vickerstaff V, Ambler G, et al. Laser in glaucoma and ocular hypertension (LiGHT) trial. Ophthalmology. 2023;130(2):139–51.

Artificial Intelligence and Optometry: Transforming Practice and Patient Care

Shivani Majithia and Sahil Thakur

1 Introduction

Artificial intelligence (AI) has emerged as a transformative force in the field of optometry, revolutionizing the way practitioners diagnose, treat, and manage ocular conditions. At the heart of AI lies machine learning (ML) and its subset, deep learning (DL), which have demonstrated remarkable capabilities in analyzing vast amounts of data to extract meaningful patterns and insights. In the realm of optometry, the advent of AI-driven technologies has been particularly notable in leveraging medical imaging data, such as retinal images and optical coherence tomography (OCT) scans. These imaging modalities provide rich information about ocular health and pathology, making them ideal inputs for AI algorithms. Moreover, the availability of large-scale datasets, such as those from initiatives like the UK Biobank, combined with advancements in computing power and chip development, has significantly lowered the barrier for developing sophisticated AI models. These datasets serve as invaluable resources for training and validating AI algorithms, enabling researchers and developers to create robust and accurate models for various optometric applications. Briefly, the development of AI models typically involves several stages, including data preprocessing, model selection, training, tuning, and testing. This iterative process aims to optimize the model's performance and generalizability across diverse datasets. Evaluating the performance of AI models then requires robust metrics that assess their accuracy, sensitivity, specificity, and predictive value. Common metrics include area under the receiver operating

S. Majithia
Education and Professional Services, Essilor Luxottica, Singapore
e-mail: shivani.majithia@essilor.com

S. Thakur (✉)
Singapore Eye Research Institute, Singapore, Singapore

Medical Affairs, Mediwhale, Seoul, South Korea

D. Shu et al. (eds.), *Current Advances in Optometry*, Current Practices in Ophthalmology, https://doi.org/10.1007/978-981-97-8140-9_11

characteristic curve (AUC-ROC), precision, recall, and F1-score. This chapter aims to provide a focused exploration of the impact of AI on optometry, with a particular emphasis on FDA-approved AI products, the transformative potential of early detection and screening, and the evolving scope of optometric practice in the AI era. While acknowledging the vast landscape of AI applications in optometry, this chapter prioritizes key themes and developments relevant to practitioners and stakeholders. It serves as a concise overview, offering insights into the current state of AI integration in optometry and outlining future directions for research and practice.

2 FDA-Approved Eye Related SaMD (Software as Medical Device) and Their Impact

In recent years, the FDA has granted approval to several AI-driven technologies designed to enhance diagnostic accuracy and streamline patient care within the field of optometry and ophthalmology. These innovations harness the power of AI, particularly ML/DL algorithms, to analyze medical imaging data and detect ocular abnormalities with high precision and efficiency. Notably, these FDA-approved AI products represent a significant milestone in the integration of AI into clinical practice, offering optometrists valuable tools for early detection and management of various ocular conditions. Notable examples include:

2.1 IDx-DR by Digital Diagnostics Inc.

IDx-DR is an autonomous AI diagnostic system authorized by the FDA for the detection of more than mild diabetic retinopathy (mtmDR) and diabetic macular edema (DME). A pivotal trial enrolled 900 subjects without a history of diabetic retinopathy (DR) at primary care clinics, comparing the system's performance to Wisconsin Fundus Photograph Reading Center (FPRC) standards. Median age was 59 years (range, 22–84 years); among participants, 47.5% were male; 16.1% were Hispanic, 83.3% were not Hispanic; 28.6% were African American, and 63.4% were not. The AI system demonstrated high sensitivity of 87.2% and specificity of 90.7%, exceeding pre-specified superiority endpoints. Furthermore, the imageability rate was 96.1%, thus showing AI's ability to bring specialty-level diagnostics to primary care settings [1].

2.2 EyeArt Automated DR Detection System by Eyenuk, Inc.

The EyeArt system has been designed to detect DR and vision-threatening diabetic retinopathy (vtDR) autonomously. A prospective multicenter cross-sectional diagnostic study, conducted from April 17, 2017, to May 30, 2018, evaluated its safety and accuracy in detecting mtmDR and vtDR in individuals with diabetes. Out of 942 consenting individuals aged 18 years or older, 893 patients (1786 eyes) met the inclusion criteria and completed the study protocol across 15 primary care and eye care facilities. The system demonstrated high sensitivity and specificity in detecting both mtmDR (sensitivity: 95.5%, specificity: 85.0%) and vtDR (sensitivity: 95.1%, specificity: 89.0%) without dilation. After correction for enrichment, the specificity for mtmDR increased to 87.8%, and both sensitivity (97.0%) and specificity (90.1%) improved for vtDR [2, 3].

These FDA-approved AI products and similar country specific derivatives have had a profound impact on the screening and diagnosis of ocular conditions, particularly DR. Their deployment in screening programs has significantly enhanced the efficiency and effectiveness of DR screening, leading to early detection and intervention in at-risk populations [4]. In many countries, AI-based solutions are starting to become integral components of national DR screening programs, offering scalable and cost-effective approaches to managing this sight-threatening complication of diabetes [4–8]. Moreover, some countries, such as Singapore and Turkey, have developed their own AI solutions tailored to their population samples, further illustrating the versatility and adaptability of AI across diverse scenarios [9–11].

3 Scope of Practice and Salient Examples of Potential AI Solutions

Optometrists serve as essential primary healthcare providers specializing in the assessment and management of the eye and visual system. Their scope of practice encompasses a wide range of services, including the evaluation of visual acuity, correction of refractive errors through prescription of glasses or contact lenses, as well as the detection, diagnosis, and treatment of various eye diseases. Additionally, optometrists play a crucial role in rehabilitating conditions affecting the visual system, offering interventions to enhance visual function and quality of life for their patients. In light of this scope of practice, this section will deal with some salient examples of AI applications that can be potentially adopted into the workflow for optometrists.

3.1 Vision Impairment

In the realm of community vision screening, there exists a pressing need for an efficient and accurate method to detect individuals requiring referral to specialized eye care centers due to vision loss associated with various eye conditions. The advent of AI and especially DL presents a promising avenue to transform this clinical referral pathway. Tham et al., in their study aimed to evaluate the efficacy of a newly developed DL algorithm in detecting disease-related visual impairment using retinal fundus images [12]. Drawing from a dataset comprising 15,175 eyes with complete data on visual acuity from the Singapore Epidemiology of Eye Diseases (SEED) Study, researchers embarked on a proof-of-concept endeavor. Initially, a single-modality DL algorithm was crafted solely from retinal photographs to discern any disease-related visual impairment, defined as eyes with major eye diseases and best-corrected visual acuity of less than 20/40, as well as moderate or worse disease-related visual impairment, indicated by eyes with disease and best-corrected visual acuity of less than 20/60. Following algorithm development, its performance was internally tested on a fresh set of 3803 eyes from the same study. Subsequently, external validation was conducted using data from three population-based studies and two clinical studies, encompassing a total of 16,993 eyes. The findings from the internal test dataset were promising, with the algorithm exhibiting an AUC of 94.2% for the detection of any disease-related visual impairment and 93.9% for moderate or worse impairment. External validation across the five test datasets demonstrated AUCs ranging from 86.6% to 93.6% for any disease-related visual impairment and between 85.9% and 93.5% for moderate or worse impairment. These results underscore the potential of this function-focused tool in promptly identifying visual impairment stemming from major eye diseases. Ultimately, such a tool holds promise for facilitating targeted and timely referrals of individuals with disease-related visual impairment from community settings to specialized eye care facilities, thereby enhancing the efficiency and effectiveness of vision care delivery.

3.2 Cataract

In the realm of optometry, where practitioners serve as primary healthcare providers for the eye and visual system, the detection and management of age-related cataracts stand as a crucial component of comprehensive eye care. Age-related cataracts, known to be the leading cause of visual impairment among older adults globally, present a significant challenge in many communities due to issues related to accessibility and availability of screening services. Despite being easily treatable through surgical intervention, a considerable number of individuals with visually significant cataracts often go undiagnosed or neglected, particularly in underserved areas where resources are limited. Traditional methods of cataract diagnosis heavily rely on slit-lamp biomicroscopy conducted by trained ophthalmologists, a process that may not be readily accessible in many communities, especially those in rural or low-income settings. This poses a significant barrier to early detection and intervention, emphasizing the need for innovative approaches to expand the reach of cataract screening. The emergence of deep learning technology and retinal photograph-based algorithms presents a promising opportunity to address these challenges, offering a more efficient and accessible means of detecting visually significant cataracts. The development and validation of a retinal photograph-based, deep learning algorithm for automated detection of visually significant cataracts were reported in a study that utilized more than 25,000 images from population-based studies [13]. In the internal test set, the AUC was 96.6%. External testing performed across three studies showed AUCs ranging from 91.6% to 96.5%. In a separate test set of 186 eyes, the algorithm's performance was compared with evaluations by four ophthalmologists. The algorithm demonstrated comparable, if not slightly superior, performance, with a sensitivity of 93.3% compared to 51.7–96.6% by ophthalmologists and a specificity of 99.0% compared to 90.7–97.9% by ophthalmologists. These findings underscore the potential of a retinal photograph-based screening tool for visually significant cataracts among older adults. The algorithm's high accuracy and sensitivity suggest its efficacy in providing more appropriate referrals to tertiary eye centers, thereby facilitating timely interventions for individuals with cataract-related visual impairment. Another study demonstrated the effectiveness of the universal AI platform that uses anterior segment photos and multilevel collaborative pattern in diagnosing and managing cataracts [14]. The research also explored an AI-based medical referral pattern aimed at enhancing collaborative efficiency and resource coverage in cataract management. The training and validation datasets were sourced from the Chinese Medical Alliance for Artificial Intelligence, covering diverse healthcare facilities and capture modes. The datasets underwent a three-step labeling process, which involved recognizing capture modes, diagnosing cataracts, and detecting referable cataracts based on etiology and severity. Additionally, the study integrated the cataract AI agent with a real-world multilevel referral pattern that involved self-monitoring at home, primary healthcare, and specialized hospital services. The results demonstrated the robust diagnostic performance of the universal AI platform and multilevel collaborative pattern across three key tasks. These tasks included capture mode recognition, cataract diagnosis (normal lens, cataract, or postoperative eye), and detection of referable cataracts. The AI platform achieved impressive AUC values ranging from 91% to over 99% in all tests. In the real-world tertiary referral pattern, the AI agent suggested referrals for 30.3% of individuals, significantly increasing the doctor-to-population service ratio by 10.2-fold compared to the traditional pattern. The findings suggest that this AI-based medical referral pattern could be extended to other common disease conditions and resource-intensive situations, offering potential benefits for public health initiatives.

3.3 Multiple Disease Detection

In recent years, deep learning systems (DLSs) have emerged as powerful tools for screening various eye diseases, including DR, glaucoma, age-related macular degeneration (AMD), and other fundus abnormalities. Several studies have evaluated the performance of DLS in detecting these diseases, highlighting their potential utility in optometry practice for early diagnosis and intervention. Ting et al., in a pioneering study, evaluated the diagnostic performance of a DLS for detecting referable diabetic retinopathy, vision-threatening diabetic retinopathy, possible glaucoma, and AMD in multiethnic populations with diabetes [15]. Using a vast dataset of retinal images, the DLS demonstrated high sensitivity and specificity for identifying these conditions, paving the way for efficient screening and referral strategies. Expanding upon this research, subsequent studies have developed DL models capable of screening multiple abnormal findings in retinal fundus images. These models were trained and validated using large datasets from diverse sources, achieving high accuracy in detecting 12 major findings, including hemorrhage, hard exudate, cotton-wool patch, drusen, and glaucomatous disc changes [16]. The DL algorithms exhibited performance comparable to human experts, demonstrating their potential as automated screening systems for various retinal abnormalities.

Further advancements in DL technology have led to the development of a deep learning platform (DLP) capable of detecting a broader range of fundus diseases and conditions [17]. This platform, trained on a comprehensive dataset of over 200,000 fundus images, demonstrated remarkable accuracy in detecting 39 classes of common fundus diseases, including DR, AMD, RVO, RAO, glaucoma, and retinal detachment. The DLP's performance rivaled that of retina specialists, suggesting its potential for use in clinical settings and population screening programs. In a real-world clinical environment, an AI-based fundus screening system also exhibited superior diagnostic effectiveness for DR, RVO, and pathological myopia (PM), achieving high sensitivity, specificity, accuracy, and predictive values [18]. This system demonstrated its clinical utility in the early detection of ocular fundus abnormalities, highlighting its role in preventing blindness through timely intervention. Collectively, these studies underscore the potential of deep learning technology in optometry practice for the comprehensive screening and detection of multiple eye diseases. By leveraging AI-based tools, optometrists can enhance their diagnostic capabilities, streamline screening processes, and improve patient outcomes through early detection and intervention.

4 Key Insights from Recent Resources

4.1 Optometry 2040

The Optometry 2040 initiative from Optometry Australia, launched in 2018, presents three distinct scenarios envisioning the future of optometry, alongside key trends shaping the profession given in Table 1.

These scenarios highlight potential trajectories for the profession, emphasizing the need for adaptation to technological advancements. Scenario 2, identified as optimal, underscores the importance of embracing collaborative and technology-enabled care delivery. Key trends identified in the report include consistently-evolving technology, enlarged scope of practice, and consumer-centric care, underscoring the importance of embracing AI and adapting practice models.

Table 1 Scenarios discussed under optometry 2040 initiative by Optometry Australia [19]

Scenario	Description
1. Optometry fails to adapt	Technological and clinical advancements render much of optometry's diagnostic work redundant, leading to underemployment and decreased salaries
2. The eye care you want—As well as the eye care you need	Optometrists become trusted guides through the eye care system, facilitated by collaborative professional-patient relationships and technology-enabled care delivery. This scenario is considered optimal for the profession
3. Optometry beyond the dark room and out of the box	Optometrists lead technological innovation, becoming 'optical scientists' and integrating with other disciplines to optimize healthcare

4.2 American Academy of Optometrists Survey

The American Academy of Optometry (AAO) survey provides insights into optometrists' perspectives on AI integration in eye care [20]. The study was conducted among 400 optometrists who completed a survey assessing perceived advantages and concerns regarding AI using a 5-point Likert scale. The majority of respondents indicated that they were familiar with AI, with approximately 66.8% reporting such familiarity. However, approximately half of optometrists expressed concerns regarding the diagnostic accuracy of AI, with around 53.0% expressing such reservations. Despite these concerns, a significant majority, accounting for 72.0% of respondents, believed that the integration of AI would enhance the practice of optometry. Furthermore, optometrists' willingness to integrate AI into their practice showed a notable increase, rising from 53.3% before the COVID-19 pandemic to 65.5% following the onset of the pandemic ($p < 0.001$).

The convergence of insights from Optometry 2040 and the AAO survey underscores the transformative potential of AI in optometric practice. While Optometry 2040 provides a visionary outlook on the future of the profession and identifies key trends shaping its trajectory, the AAO survey offers a snapshot of current perceptions and attitudes toward AI integration among optometrists. Together, these resources offer valuable perspectives on the opportunities and challenges associated with AI adoption in optometry, highlighting the importance of strategic planning, education, and collaboration to navigate the evolving landscape of eye care delivery. As optometry moves toward an AI-enabled future, it is essential for practitioners to embrace innovation while upholding core principles of patient-centered care and professional excellence.

5 LLMs and Foundation Models: The Next Frontier

Large language models (LLMs) have emerged as powerful tools with significant potential to transform various aspects of optometry practice. These models, such as ChatGPT, Google Bard (now Gemini), and Bing Chat, are trained on vast datasets and possess human-like text generation capabilities. In the context of optometry, LLMs can play a crucial role in enhancing diagnosis, treatment, patient care, and expanding the scope of practice. One area where LLMs demonstrate promise is in aiding during optometric exams and consultations. For example, eye-specific LLMs, specifically designed for ophthalmic applications, have been evaluated for their performance in assisting with the Fellowship of Royal College of Ophthalmologists (FRCOphth) exams [21]. These models have shown varying degrees of accuracy in answering multiple-choice questions related to ophthalmology, with differences observed among different LLM-chatbots. This underscores the importance of continued research and refinement to optimize the performance of LLMs in supporting eye related education and assessment. In addition to assisting with clinical decision-making, LLMs can also facilitate patient communication and education [22]. ChatGPT, for instance, can be integrated into virtual consultations, allowing patients to ask questions and receive personalized responses regarding their eye health concerns. This not only enhances patient engagement but also promotes proactive management of ocular conditions.

Moreover, foundation models like RETFound represent a significant advancement in leveraging AI for eye care. RETFound, developed by Moorfields Eye Hospital and University College London, is an AI foundation model specifically trained 1.6 million unlabeled retinal images by means of self-supervised learning [23]. This model has demonstrated the ability to detect sight-threatening eye diseases and even predict systemic health challenges such as heart attacks, stroke, and Parkinson's disease. One notable advantage is their ability to reduce the need for extensive dataset collection. Unlike conventional AI models that require massive amounts of labeled data for training, foundation models leverage self-supervised learning techniques to learn from unannotated or minimally labeled data. This means that RETFound can extract valuable insights from a relatively small dataset of retinal images, thereby streamlining the data collection process and reducing the burden on healthcare institutions to amass large datasets. Moreover, foundation models enable faster and more customized development of AI solutions through techniques such as few-shot and zero-shot learning. *Few-shot learning* allows models like RETFound to adapt to new tasks or domains with minimal labeled examples, making it possible to tailor the model to specific clinical applications rapidly. For example, RETFound can be fine-tuned to detect rare or emerging eye diseases using only a handful of annotated images, accelerating the development of novel diagnostic tools. *Zero-shot learning* takes this concept further by enabling the model to generalize to tasks it has never encountered before. This capability is particularly valuable for rare diseases, where clinicians may not have enough data or samples to train models. With RETFound, optometrists can leverage the model's pretrained knowledge to address new challenges without the need for additional data collection or model retraining. Furthermore, foundation models like RETFound democratize AI by making state-of-the-art technology accessible to a broader audience. Traditionally, AI development has been confined to research labs and tech giants with the resources to collect and process massive datasets [24]. However, with the advent of foundation models, even smaller clinics or research institutions can harness the power of AI to improve patient care. By providing open access to pretrained models and resources for model adaptation, solutions like RETFound empower clinicians and researchers to innovate and develop AI solutions tailored to their unique needs and patient populations.

However, the integration of LLMs and foundation models into current practice necessitates upskilling and adaptation among optometrists. Continuous learning and development programs are essential to ensure that practitioners are proficient in leveraging and using AI tools effectively. Strategies for embracing AI, such as incorporating LLM-driven chatbots into practice workflows and collaborating with technologists to develop specialized models, are vital for optimizing the benefits of AI integration. Overall, the impact of LLMs and foundation models in vision science extends beyond conventional diagnostic and treatment paradigms. These models hold the potential to revolutionize the way we deliver care, interact with patients, and contribute to advancements in ocular health.

References

1. Abràmoff MD, Lavin PT, Birch M, Shah N, Folk JC. Pivotal trial of an autonomous AI-based diagnostic system for detection of diabetic retinopathy in primary care offices. NPJ Digit Med. 2018;1(1):39.
2. Ipp E, Liljenquist D, Bode B, Shah VN, Silverstein S, Regillo CD, et al. Pivotal evaluation of an artificial intelligence system for autonomous detection of referrable and vision-threatening diabetic retinopathy. JAMA Netw Open. 2021;4(11):e2134254.
3. Lim JI, Regillo CD, Sadda SR, Ipp E, Bhaskaranand M, Ramachandra C, et al. Artificial intelligence detection of diabetic retinopathy: subgroup comparison of the EyeArt system with ophthalmologists' dilated examinations. Ophthalmol Sci. 2023;3(1):100228.
4. Heydon P, Egan C, Bolter L, Chambers R, Anderson J, Aldington S, et al. Prospective evaluation of an artificial intelligence-enabled algorithm for automated diabetic retinopathy screening of 30,000 patients. Br J Ophthalmol. 2021;105(5):723–8.
5. Cleland CR, Bascaran C, Makupa W, Shilio B, Sandi FA, Philippin H, et al. Artificial intelligence-supported diabetic retinopathy screening in Tanzania: rationale and design of a randomised controlled trial. BMJ Open. 2024;14(1):e075055.
6. Ruamviboonsuk P, Tiwari R, Sayres R, Nganthavee V, Hemarat K, Kongprayoon A, et al. Real-time diabetic retinopathy screening by deep learning in a multisite national screening programme: a prospective interventional cohort study. Lancet Digit Health. 2022;4(4):e235–e44.
7. Arenas-Cavalli JT, Abarca I, Rojas-Contreras M, Bernuy F, Donoso R. Clinical validation of an artificial intelligence-based diabetic retinopathy screening tool for a national health system. Eye. 2022;36(1):78–85.
8. Huang XM, Yang BF, Zheng WL, Liu Q, Xiao F, Ouyang PW, et al. Cost-effectiveness of artificial intelligence screening for diabetic retinopathy in rural China. BMC Health Serv Res. 2022;22(1):260.
9. MOH | News Highlights 2024 [updated 2024/03/23/]. Available from: https://www.moh.gov.sg/news-highlights/details/efficacy-of-the-selena-system.
10. Wong DCS, Kiew G, Jeon S, Ting D. Singapore eye lesions analyzer (SELENA): the deep learning system for retinal diseases. In: Grzybowski A, editor. Artificial intelligence in ophthalmology. Cham: Springer International Publishing; 2021. p. 177–85.
11. Doğan ME, Bilgin AB, Sari R, Bulut M, Akar Y, Aydemir M. Head to head comparison of diagnostic performance of three non-mydriatic cameras for diabetic retinopathy screening with artificial intelligence. Eye. 2024;38:1694–701.
12. Tham Y-C, Anees A, Zhang L, Goh JHL, Rim TH, Nusinovici S, et al. Referral for disease-related visual impairment using retinal photograph-based deep learning: a proof-of-concept, model development study. Lancet Digit Health. 2021;3(1):e29–40.
13. Tham Y-C, Goh JHL, Anees A, Lei X, Rim TH, Chee M-L, et al. Detecting visually significant cataract using retinal photograph-based deep learning. Nat Aging. 2022;2(3):264–71.
14. Wu X, Huang Y, Liu Z, Lai W, Long E, Zhang K, et al. Universal artificial intelligence platform for collaborative management of cataracts. Br J Ophthalmol. 2019;103(11):1553.
15. Ting DSW, Cheung CY-L, Lim G, Tan GSW, Quang ND, Gan A, et al. Development and validation of a deep learning system for diabetic retinopathy and related eye diseases using retinal images from multiethnic populations with diabetes. JAMA. 2017;318(22):2211–23.
16. Son J, Shin JY, Kim HD, Jung KH, Park KH, Park SJ. Development and validation of deep learning models for screening multiple abnormal findings in retinal fundus images. Ophthalmology. 2020;127(1):85–94.
17. Cen L-P, Ji J, Lin J-W, Ju S-T, Lin H-J, Li T-P, et al. Automatic detection of 39 fundus diseases and conditions in retinal photographs using deep neural networks. Nat Commun. 2021;12(1):4828.
18. Cao S, Zhang R, Jiang A, Kuerban M, Wumaier A, Wu J, et al. Application effect of an artificial intelligence-based fundus screening system: evaluation in a clinical setting and population screening. Biomed Eng Online. 2023;22(1):38.

19. Optometry 2040—Optometry Australia. (Accessed from: https://www.optometry.org.au/about-us/our-current-focus/optometry-2040/).
20. Scanzera AC, Shorter E, Kinnaird C, Valikodath N, Al-Khaled T, Cole E, et al. Optometrist's perspectives of artificial intelligence in eye care. J Optom. 2022;15(Suppl 1):S91–s7.
21. Raimondi R, Tzoumas N, Salisbury T, Di Simplicio S, Romano MR, Bommireddy T, et al. Comparative analysis of large language models in the royal college of ophthalmologists fellowship exams. Eye. 2023;37(17):3530–3.
22. Huang AS, Hirabayashi K, Barna L, Parikh D, Pasquale LR. Assessment of a large language model's responses to questions and cases about glaucoma and retina management. JAMA Ophthalmol. 2024;142:371–5.
23. Zhou Y, Chia MA, Wagner SK, Ayhan MS, Williamson DJ, Struyven RR, et al. A foundation model for generalizable disease detection from retinal images. Nature. 2023;622(7981):156–63.
24. Cheng C-Y, Soh ZD, Majithia S, Thakur S, Rim TH, Tham YC, et al. Big data in ophthalmology. Asia-Pac J Ophthalmol. 2020;9(4):291–8.

MIX
Papier aus verantwortungsvollen Quellen
Paper from responsible sources
FSC® C105338

FSC
www.fsc.org

If you have any concerns about our products,
you can contact us on
ProductSafety@springernature.com

In case Publisher is established outside the EU,
the EU authorized representative is:
Springer Nature Customer Service Center GmbH
Europaplatz 3, 69115 Heidelberg, Germany

Printed by Libri Plureos GmbH
in Hamburg, Germany